The Night Is Normal Workbook

. . .

ALICIA BRITT CHOLE

AN HONEST JOURNEY THROUGH SPIRITUAL PAIN

THE
NIGHT
IS
NORMAL

WORKBOOK

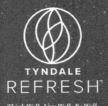

TYNDALE
REFRESH

Think Well. Live Well. Be Well.

Visit Tyndale online at tyndale.com.

Visit the author online at https://aliciachole.com.

Tyndale, Tyndale's quill logo, *Tyndale Refresh,* and the Tyndale Refresh logo are registered trademarks of Tyndale House Ministries. Tyndale Refresh is a nonfiction imprint of Tyndale House Publishers, Carol Stream, Illinois.

The Night Is Normal Workbook: An Honest Journey through Spiritual Pain

Copyright © 2024 by Dr. Alicia Britt Chole. All rights reserved.

Cover illustration of intersecting circles by Lindsey Bergsma. Copyright © Tyndale House Ministries. All rights reserved.

Cover photograph of stars by Guille Pozzi on Unsplash.com

Author photograph by Randy Bacon, Copyright © 2022. All Rights Reserved.

Designed by Lindsey Bergsma

Scripture quotations are taken from the Holy Bible, *New International Version,*® *NIV.*® Copyright © 1973, 1978, 1984 by Biblica, Inc.® Used by permission. All rights reserved worldwide.

For information about special discounts for bulk purchases, please contact Tyndale House Publishers at csresponse@tyndale.com, or call 1-855-277-9400.

ISBN 978-1-4964-7828-3

Printed in the United States of America

30	29	28	27	26	25	24
7	6	5	4	3	2	1

Contents

How to Use This Workbook

Reading is a good thing. Discussing is a great thing. And applying what one has read and discussed can enrich the future of generations. That's why I'm offering this workbook and its accompanying teaching videos. I hope these additional offerings will help you navigate your nights of spiritual pain with a sturdy hope.

The fifty-two short chapters of *The Night Is Normal* are organized in four parts. This workbook devotes two sessions to each part via a chapter-by-chapter offering formatted in three components: *Reflect* upon the chapter's content, *Study* the Scriptures, and *Respond* personally to the chapter's principles.

Several possibilities exist for using this workbook in groups.

1. For a sixty-minute group time, encourage participants to read the chapters and do the *Study* and *Respond* sections beforehand. Then, together, watch the video and go through the *Reflect* sections.
2. For a ninety-minute group time, encourage participants to read the chapters and do the *Respond* sections beforehand. Then, together, watch the video and go through the *Reflect* and *Study* sections.
3. Whatever your time frame, feel free to not do it all. Without question, for sustainable fruit from this study, quality of thought and application outweighs quantity of questions completed.

If you're using the workbook as an individual or with a friend, pause after reading each chapter in *The Night Is Normal* to go through each week's *Reflect*, *Study*, and *Respond* sections. Feel free to add or subtract the videos as time permits.

May these words help us all lose our fear of the dark,

Alicia
@aliciabrittchole
www.aliciachole.com

Navigating the Night

Now the earth was formless and empty, darkness was over the surface of the deep, and the Spirit of God was hovering over the waters. And God said, "Let there be light," and there was light. God saw that the light was good, and he separated the light from the darkness. God called the light "day," and the darkness he called "night." And there was evening, and there was morning—the first day.

GENESIS 1:2-5

Chapter 1

. . .

FACING THE STORM TOGETHER

REFLECT

1. What gift did Alicia's dad give to her on their many front porches? (See pages 3–4.)

   _____

   _____

   _____

   _____

2. Encouraging readers to bring their questions with them, Alicia says, "I view their primary purpose as _____ _____ instead of _____ _____"
   (see page 6).

3. How comfortable are you with asking God sincere questions?

   _____

   _____

   _____

4. "God has not changed. But our understanding of what it means to follow Him has undergone an alarming mutation from the dual toxins of mistaking emotions for devotion and viewing abundance as proof of obedience" (page 6). Do you see evidence of these "dual toxins" in your culture?

   _____

   _____

   _____

   _____

STUDY

Consider Psalm 139:7-12:

Where can I go from your Spirit? Where can I flee from your presence? If I go up to the heavens, you are there; if I make my bed in the depths, you are there. If I rise on the wings of the dawn, if I settle on the far side of the sea, even there your hand will guide me, your right hand will hold me fast. If I say, "Surely the darkness will hide me and the light become night around me," even the darkness will not be dark to you; the night will shine like the day, for darkness is as light to you.

1. In the passage, underline the places in which the psalmist knew God would be with him.

2. Which of these locations gives you the most comfort?

_____

_____

_____

_____

_____

3. Spend a moment picturing God right next to you. His proximity is your theological reality. He is with you every second of every day. How can that reality affect your perspective today?

_____

_____

_____

_____

_____

> STORMS ARE SURVIVABLE
> WHEN WE VIEW THEM AS RELATIONAL.
> THE NIGHT IS FILLED WITH HOLY INVITATIONS
> TO GROW OUR LOVE FOR GOD.

RESPOND

1. What storms are you currently facing?

   _____

   _____

   _____

   _____

   _____

2. Did you have someone in your life who, like Alicia's dad, was present in the midst of night-storms?

   _____

   _____

   _____

   _____

   _____

3. Whether your response is a pain-filled "no" or a grateful "yes," in faith, picture yourself on a porch with Father God near. Use the space below to write an honest prayer to God.

   _____

   _____

   _____

   _____

   _____

   _____

   _____

> BRING ANY UNCERTAINTY,
> FRUSTRATION, AND PAIN WITH YOU.
> DENIAL—HOWEVER POLITE OR WELL-INTENDED—
> HAS NO REGENERATIVE POWER.

Chapter 2

. . .

NIGHT-FAITH

REFLECT

1. Is Alicia's park-bench experience familiar to you? If so, what feelings did you have when it seemed as though your grip on faith was failing?

_____

_____

_____

_____

2. On page 11, Alicia points out that "night was one of the original residents of Eden." What difference does it make to you personally that "night-faith was as much a part of God's 'in the beginning' goodness as day-faith"?

_____

_____

_____

_____

STUDY

Read Acts 9:3-6, 8-9:

> As he neared Damascus on his journey, suddenly a light from heaven flashed around him. He fell to the ground and heard a voice say to him, "Saul, Saul, why do you persecute me?" "Who are you, Lord?" Saul asked. "I am Jesus, whom you are persecuting," he replied. "Now get up and go into the city, and you will be told what you must do." . . . Saul got up from the ground, but when he opened his eyes he could see nothing. So

they led him by the hand into Damascus. For three days he was blind, and did not eat or drink anything.

The word translated "light" is *phos*. According to Spiros Zodhiates, this word is "used metaphorically with reference to God (1 John 1:5), Jesus Christ (John 1:7-9), spiritual illumination (Matthew 4:16; Luke 2:32; John 1:4-5; Acts 13:47; Romans 2:19)."[*]

A close encounter with Jesus left Saul in darkness for three days. In what ways might darkness have been a gift for Saul in the earliest moments of his journey with Jesus?

_____

_____

_____

_____

RESPOND

"What if avoiding the night is sabotaging the health of our souls?" (page 12). Personally, what has been the cost of avoidance in your life?

_____

_____

_____

_____

_____

_____

> IT SEEMS THAT NIGHT-FAITH WAS AS MUCH A PART
> OF GOD'S "IN THE BEGINNING" GOODNESS AS DAY-FAITH.
> PRE-SIN, PRE-FALL, PRE-CURSE, AND PRE-DRAMA,
> NIGHT WAS ONE OF THE ORIGINAL RESIDENTS OF EDEN.

---

[*] Lexical Aids to the New Testament, compiled and edited by Spiros Zodhiates, ThD, *Hebrew-Greek Key Word Study Bible: New International Version* (Chattanooga, TN: AMG Publishers, 1996):1685.

Chapter 3

. . .

THAT STARTLING "POP"

REFLECT

1. Write down the two definitions of *disillusionment* Alicia offers on pages 16–17.

2. What gains have you experienced from spiritual pain?

> DISILLUSIONMENT IS NOT ALL LOSS.
> WHEN WE ARE DISILLUSIONED, LOSS IS MAKING
> WAY WITHIN US FOR A POWERFUL GAIN.

STUDY

Read Romans 8:28:

And we know that in all things God works for the good of those who love him, who have been called according to his purpose.

1. Paul knew darkness, both spiritually and physically. The first darkness led him into hate. The second, into love. Throughout Chapters 3–5, Alicia is reframing disillusionment for us definitionally, biblically, and historically. In what ways have you already seen God working in your disillusionment for your good?

_____

_____

_____

2. Review Alicia's illustration of the balloon popping. How might this shift in perspective affect your daily life?

_____

_____

_____

RESPOND

Pause to ask God to help "the soul-deep sadness of disillusionment" to challenge and purify your belief in Him (page 17).

_____

_____

_____

_____

LIVING FAITH CAN NEVER BE REDUCED TO LIFELESS FORMULAS.
FORMULAS GUT FAITH OF RELATIONSHIP.
AND IF FAITH IS ANYTHING, IT IS RELATIONAL.

Chapter 4

. . .

WHAT'S IN A WORD, PART ONE

REFLECT

1. Peruse the words and phrases presented in the table running parallel throughout chapter 4. What conclusions can you draw from this overview of 1,500 years of terms that have been used to capture the concept of spiritual pain?

2. Share any way in which your nights have strengthened your relationship with God.

STUDY

Read Job 42:1-3:

> Then Job replied to the LORD: "I know that you can do all things; no plan of yours can be thwarted. You asked, 'Who is this that obscures my counsel without knowledge?' Surely I spoke of things I did not understand, things too wonderful for me to know."

What reality about God did Job gain through his dark night?

_____

_____

_____

_____

_____

_____

RESPOND

Offer this simple prayer to God:

Savior, my head knows that You are with me in the night as much as in the day. But my heart is sometimes slower to believe that this reality is true. Like Job, strengthen me to be honest with You about the spiritual pain in my life. And like Job, open my eyes to see You more accurately through every night.

> YOUR NIGHTS, THOUGH NORMAL, ARE NOT ETERNAL.
> AND WITHIN EACH ONE IS AN INVITATION
> TO STRENGTHEN YOUR RELATIONSHIP WITH GOD.

Chapter 5

. . .

WHAT'S IN A WORD, PART TWO

REFLECT

1. In your own words, how is disillusionment distinct from cynicism, skepticism, and despair? (See pages 26–31.)

2. Which, if any, of these states are you naturally more vulnerable to?

3. On page 30, Alicia states that the loss we experience in the night gives way to

STUDY

Read Exodus 20:20-21:

> Moses said to the people, "Do not be afraid. God has come to test you, so that the fear of God will be with you to keep you from sinning." The people remained at a distance, while Moses approached the thick darkness where God was.

The Hebrew word translated here as "thick darkness" also appears in Deuteronomy 4:11; 5:22; Job 22:13; 38:9; Psalm 97:2; Isaiah 60:2; and Ezekiel 34:12. Read (or take turns reading) these passages. What do you notice about this type of darkness, within which Moses met God?

_____

_____

_____

_____

_____

_____

RESPOND

"If we do not normalize the night in the life of faith, we can easily mistake spiritual darkness for spiritual death" (page 30). Slow down enough to honestly ask yourself if you've mistaken darkness for death in your spiritual life. Write any reflections below.

_____

_____

_____

_____

_____

_____

_____

> OUR WIRED AGE IS FERTILE SOIL
> FOR THE PROLIFERATION OF CYNICISM.
> HIDDEN SAFELY BEHIND SCREENS, OUR GENERATION CAN
> FIND FAULT EFFORTLESSLY AND ANONYMOUSLY.

PART ONE

• • •

Navigating
the Night

WEEK 2, CHAPTERS 6–10

Now we see but a poor reflection as in a mirror; then we shall see face to face.
Now I know in part; then I shall know fully, even as I am fully known.

1 CORINTHIANS 13:12

Chapter 6

. . .

A RELATIONAL CYCLE

REFLECT

1. For Alicia, the messy parts of Scripture increased her "confidence in its authenticity" (page 32). Why? Do you agree or disagree with her logic?

_____

_____

_____

_____

2. Give an example from your own life of "joyful anticipation."

_____

_____

_____

3. Draw Alicia's illustration of the cycle of relationship from page 36 and then respond to the question she asks: "Can you see our generation stuck in this cycle?"

4. In your generation, do you see evidence of the following? "Without certainty that disillusionment is a well-traveled path *within* faith, we assume that experiencing disillusionment somehow means that we have moved outside the faith" (page 37).

_____

_____

_____

_____

_____

> IN THE ABSENCE OF A THEOLOGICAL FRAMEWORK WITHIN
> WHICH TO RECOGNIZE THE NIGHT AS NORMAL IN OUR FAITH,
> WE MISTAKE THE NIGHT FOR NOTHINGNESS.

STUDY

Read Hebrews 11:35b-39:

Others were tortured and refused to be released, so that they might gain a better resurrection. Some faced jeers and flogging, while still others were chained and put in prison. They were stoned; they were sawed in two; they were put to death by the sword. They went about in sheepskins and goatskins, destitute, persecuted and mistreated—the world was not worthy of them. They wandered in deserts and mountains, and in caves and holes in the ground. These were all commended for their faith.

1. Consider the stories of these "others" in the Hebrews 11 hall of faith. What spiritual pain must they have known? What questions must they have asked?

_____

_____

_____

_____

_____

2. What do you think strengthened them to not bail in their faith during such disillusioning days and endings?

_____

_____

_____

_____

_____

_____

RESPOND

"In disillusionment, shiny (yet sometimes shallow) ideals are lost, as deeper (yet initially duller) reality is gained" (page 37). Think of someone you know who has lost some shiny ideals. How can you encourage them today?

_____

_____

_____

_____

_____

_____

_____

> DISILLUSIONMENT IS EVIDENCE OF GROWTH,
> NOT DECAY.

Chapter 7

. . .

BETWEEN ILLUSION
AND REALITY

REFLECT

1. What reasoning does Alicia offer to normalize the presence of illusions in our faith-walk? (See pages 39–40.)

2. How has your understanding of God grown since you first committed to follow Him?

3. On page 40, Alicia speaks of our tendency to add on to what we "know in part" (1 Corinthians 13:12). Does this tendency feel familiar to you?

STUDY

Read Proverbs 3:5-6:

Trust in the LORD with all your heart and lean not on your own understanding; in all your ways acknowledge him, and he will make your paths straight.

1. Write this familiar passage in your own words.

   _____

   _____

   _____

2. On page 42, Alicia states, "When in pain, we have to decide what we love more and what our faith is really in. Is our love and faith in God or in our understanding? (The former will always be too big for the latter.)" What helpful steps have you taken when life has tempted you to place your faith in your own understanding instead of in God?

   _____

   _____

   _____

   _____

RESPOND

"'Only let us live up to what we have already attained' (Philippians 3:16). What a relief! We do not have to hold earlier versions of ourselves accountable for what our current version barely now knows!" (page 41). Take a deep breath and give yourself grace to still be growing.

   _____

   _____

   _____

   _____

WHEN IN PAIN, WE HAVE TO DECIDE WHAT
WE LOVE MORE AND WHAT OUR FAITH IS REALLY IN.
IS OUR LOVE AND FAITH IN GOD OR IN OUR UNDERSTANDING?
(THE FORMER WILL ALWAYS BE TOO BIG FOR THE LATTER.)

Chapter 8

· · ·

THE UPWARD PULL
OF LOVE

REFLECT

1. What is the surprising alternative to bailing that Alicia introduces to her illustration in Chapter 8? How does she define it? (See pages 45–46.)

_____

_____

_____

_____

2. "Sometimes I picture the upward pull of God's love as a divine magnet, lifting me to my true home. When we are disillusioned and choose love, our minds are drawn heavenward, and our souls move Godward" (page 47). What works against our need to choose love when disillusioned?

_____

_____

_____

_____

_____

STUDY

Read Luke 7:17-19, 22a, 23:

> This news about Jesus spread throughout Judea and the surrounding country. John's disciples told him about all these things. Calling two of them, he sent them to the Lord to ask, "Are you the one who was to come, or should we expect someone else?" . . . So he

replied to the messengers, "Go back and report to John what you have seen and heard. . . . Blessed is the man who does not fall away on account of me."

1. John the Baptist sent this message to Jesus from within a dark prison cell. In what ways might John have felt disillusioned with Jesus?

_____

_____

_____

_____

2. Imagine yourself as John receiving Jesus' response: "Blessed is the man who does not fall away on account of me." Rephrase this sentence in your own words.

_____

_____

_____

_____

3. How might Jesus' message have kept John from bailing in his final night of life?

_____

_____

_____

_____

_____

_____

_____

LIKE FAITH AND HOPE, LOVE IS NOT MERELY AN EMOTION. LOVE IS MORE LIKE A MUSCLE THAT BECOMES STRONGER THE MORE YOU CHOOSE TO USE IT.

RESPOND

1. Draw the completed illustration from page 45.

2. Now consider this image in light of the following statement: "This is the treasure refined through disillusionment—a love that keeps increasing in strength and stability with each cycle as we lose more illusions, gain more reality, and choose again and again not to bail" (page 47).

3. Ask God to strengthen you to choose the way of love in the midst of your pain.

_____

_____

_____

_____

_____

_____

_____

_____

Chapter 9

. . .

A CHOICE IN THE DARK

REFLECT

1. "In the night, God's presence in the darkness frees us to trust more, even when we know less" (page 48). What is our natural instinct when the lights go out in a room, leaving us in darkness?

_____

_____

_____

_____

2. Have you ever preferred an illusion over a reality because the illusion seemed less painful?

_____

_____

_____

_____

3. Discuss the ways in which Jesus is so much more than anything else you could reach for in the dark.

_____

_____

_____

_____

_____

_____

4. Describe how "commitment—not certainty" carried Alicia upward into love in the adoption process. (See page 51.)

_____

_____

_____

_____

5. How can deliverance from self-protection come in the form of disillusionment? (See page 56.)

_____

_____

_____

_____

_____

_____

_____

ANSWERS DO NOT CARRY US THROUGH THE NIGHT; LOVE DOES.

STUDY

Read Matthew 4:18-20:

> As Jesus was walking beside the Sea of Galilee, he saw two brothers, Simon called Peter and his brother Andrew. They were casting a net into the lake, for they were fishermen. "Come, follow me," Jesus said, "and I will make you fishers of men." At once they left their nets and followed him.

1. Picture Peter hearing this call and choosing to follow Jesus. Where might Peter have thought in the beginning that Jesus' "follow" would lead him?

_____

_____

_____

_____

2. How about you? When you first said "yes" to following Jesus, did you have thoughts about where that would lead you?

_____

_____

_____

3. How have you found the strength to keep following Jesus when you had no idea where He was leading you?

_____

_____

_____

_____

RESPOND

1. Imagine God's love pulling you upward. Spend a few minutes thinking about how saying yes to that upward pull is an image of commitment to God.

2. "Our trust muscles get more of a workout in the night (when we cannot self-guide) than in the day (when we think we can)" (page 49). In prayer, thank God for the workout of the nights in your life.

_____

_____

_____

_____

_____

_____

> THROUGHOUT THE GOSPELS, JESUS' "FOLLOW ME" NEVER INCLUDED GPS COORDINATES. FOLLOWING HAS ALWAYS BEEN MORE ABOUT *WHO* WE ARE *WITH* THAN *WHERE* WE ARE *GOING*."

Chapter 10

. . .

A SPIRITUAL EXFOLIATE

REFLECT

1. How did Alicia relate the story of the dog bites to the concept of spiritual self-protection? (See pages 53–54.)

_____

_____

2. Respond to the question on page 55: "Have you ever been so spiritually disappointed that you distanced your heart from hope or dialed back your personalization of God's love?"

_____

_____

3. Have you ever used an exfoliate? If so, for what purpose?

_____

_____

4. In what way is disillusionment a spiritual exfoliate? (See page 56.)

_____

_____

STUDY

Read Genesis 3:7-10:

Then the eyes of both of them were opened, and they realized they were naked; so they sewed fig leaves together and made coverings for themselves. Then the man and his wife heard the sound of the Lord God as he was walking in the garden in the cool of the day, and they hid from the LORD God among the trees of the garden. But the LORD God called to the man, "Where are you?" He answered, "I heard you in the garden, and I was afraid because I was naked; so I hid."

1. Why did Adam and Eve hide?

_____

2. Where and how did they hide?

_____

3. How logical was their (and our) effort to hide from God?

_____

_____

RESPOND

1. Since hiding from God is, well, impossible, why do His followers still hide? What do you think we're really hiding from?

_____

_____

_____

_____

2. Invite God to remove any layers of self-protection that are hindering your experience of the fullness of His great love.

_____

_____

> DISRUPTING THE ENEMY'S AGENDA OF CREATING DISTANCE IS ONE OF THE SACRED WORKS OF THE NIGHT. THERE, IN THE DARKNESS, OUR DEEPEST SELF-PROTECTIVE DEFAULTS ARE EXPOSED, EXAMINED, AND ABANDONED THROUGH SPIRITUAL PAIN.

PART TWO

• • •

Disillusionment with God

WEEK 3, CHAPTERS 11–18

As the deer pants for streams of water, so my soul pants for you, O God.

PSALM 42:1

Chapter 11

. . .

YELLOW JACKETS

REFLECT

Recount the story of the yellow jackets. As you feel comfortable, share times in which you've echoed Keona's question about pain in the life of someone you loved.

_____

_____

_____

_____

STUDY

Read Mark 14:35-36:

Going a little farther, he fell to the ground and prayed that if possible the hour might pass from him. "Abba, Father," he said, "everything is possible for you. Take this cup from me. Yet not what I will, but what you will."

1. Earlier, Jesus told the Twelve, "With God all things are possible" in response to their question, "Who then can be saved?" (see Matthew 19:25-26). What do you think Jesus was referring to when He asked for "the hour" to pass and "this cup" to be taken from Him?

_____

_____

_____

_____

2. To the extent you feel comfortable, share any hours or cups you wish would pass out of your life currently.

_____

_____

_____

_____

RESPOND

1. Alicia speaks of the freedom to ask hard questions. Was this freedom emphasized in your childhood?

_____

_____

_____

_____

2. In God's presence, be free to ask hard questions. Write down and then speak out loud any doubt or disillusionment that you may have been hiding from yourself and from Him.

_____

_____

_____

_____

_____

_____

_____

> AS FAR AS POTENTIAL SPIRITUAL HEALTH,
> THERE IS A SIGNIFICANT DIFFERENCE BETWEEN
> *NEVER QUESTIONING GOD* AND
> *NEVER BEING ALLOWED TO QUESTION GOD.*

Chapter 12

. . .

WHAT GOD WANTS

REFLECT

How did you feel when you read the following? "I thought God and I were working toward the same goal: ending the pain. Instead, 'success,' from His viewpoint, had less to do with my ability to change the scenery and more to do with my continued commitment to His company" (page 65).

_____

_____

_____

_____

STUDY

Read Romans 5:3-5:

Not only so, but we also rejoice in our sufferings, because we know that suffering produces perseverance; perseverance, character; and character, hope. And hope does not disappoint us, because God has poured out his love into our hearts by the Holy Spirit, whom he has given us.

1. Use your own words to describe the changes that suffering can bring.

_____

_____

_____

2. Do you think that these changes are automatic? Why or why not?

_____

_____

_____

_____

_____

_____

RESPOND

Alicia confesses that "In the night, my treasure was *fixing things* through *figuring out things*. God's treasure was my *follow*" (page 66). Ask God to reveal to you any areas in which you've placed your hope more in figuring things out than in following Jesus.

_____

_____

_____

_____

_____

_____

_____

_____

_____

> WHEN IT COMES TO RELATIONAL PAIN (WITH GOD, WITH OUR FAITH, AND WITH OTHERS OF FAITH), THE PREFACE TO OUR DISILLUSIONMENT IS RARELY KNOWN IN FULL. THERE ARE FORCES IN PLAY THAT ARE BEYOND OUR VIEW.

Chapter 13

. . .

SOMETHING OLD

REFLECT

"Panting is caused when something is so essential that its absence leaves us in desperate need. Panting is about scarcity, not plenty; about mourning drought, not celebrating outpouring; about malady, not miracles" (page 69).

Recall a time in which you have truly panted for God.

_____

_____

_____

_____

STUDY

Read Psalm 42:1-3:

As the deer pants for streams of water, so my soul pants for you, O God. My soul thirsts for God, for the living God. When can I go and meet with God? My tears have been my food day and night, while men say to me all day long, "Where is your God?"

1. Have you ever been so parched that you were physically panting? If so, when?

_____

_____

_____

2. Instead of picturing a deer by a bubbling brook lapping water, picture a deer panting for water that can't be found. What adjectives would you use to describe that situation?

_____

_____

_____

3. What had been the psalmist's food day and night?

_____

_____

_____

4. And what did those nearby feed him?

_____

_____

_____

RESPOND

Psalm 42:8 reads, "By day the LORD directs his love, at night his song is with me—a prayer to the God of my life."

Ask God to give you a night-song. Listen, and if a hymn or song or verse comes to mind, write its name or reference below.

_____

_____

_____

THIS ANCIENT JOURNEY THROUGH THE NIGHT
IS SO IMPORTANT TO GOD THAT HE INSPIRED WRITERS
TO INCLUDE IN HIS WORD STORY UPON STORY
OF THE PAINFUL GAINING OF REALITY.

Chapter 14

. . .

SOMETHING NEW, PART ONE

REFLECT

1. What biblical examples of disillusionment with Jesus' timing are offered in this chapter? (See pages 72–74.)

_____

_____

_____

2. What was the point of the illustration about April weather in North Dakota and Texas? (See pages 74–75.)

_____

_____

_____

3. Has there ever been a gap in perspective between you and a child in your life? If so, tell the story and what factors may have contributed to the differences in expectations.

_____

_____

_____

4. Are there any similarities between that story and when you have felt that God is late or negligent in your life?

_____

_____

_____

STUDY

Read Mark 4:35-38:

> That day when evening came, he said to his disciples, "Let us go over to the other side."
> Leaving the crowd behind, they took him along, just as he was, in the boat. There were
> also other boats with him. A furious squall came up, and the waves broke over the boat,
> so that it was nearly swamped. Jesus was in the stern, sleeping on a cushion. The disciples
> woke him and said to him, "Teacher, don't you care if we drown?"

As you read this passage, circle the descriptors of circumstance. Then imagine that you are one of
the disciples in the boat during the sudden storm. See Jesus sleeping peacefully. See the waves break-
ing over the boat violently. What feelings and questions do you think the disciples might have had
about Jesus and His timing?

_____

_____

_____

_____

_____

RESPOND

Looking over your life, when have you voiced to God Mary and Martha's painful cry recorded
in John 11:21 and 32 of "If you had been here . . ."?

_____

_____

_____

_____

_____

WE SKIP TO THE MIRACLES IN THE SCRIPTURES AND EXPECT
TO SKIP TO THE MIRACLES IN OUR LIVES. THE SPACE IN BETWEEN,
HOWEVER, IS WHERE LOVE VIA COMMITMENT GROWS.

Chapter 15

. . .

SOMETHING NEW, PART TWO

REFLECT

Jesus' timing, words, and ways often disillusioned His followers. Of these three areas, which do you struggle with the most?

_____

_____

_____

STUDY

Read Matthew 17:22-23:

When they came together in Galilee, he said to them, "The Son of Man is going to be betrayed into the hands of men. They will kill him, and on the third day he will be raised to life." And the disciples were filled with grief.

1. Read the surrounding context of this passage. What happened right before it? Right after it?

_____

_____

_____

2. Why do you think that the disciples "were filled with grief"?

_____

_____

_____

_____

RESPOND

Prayerfully journal a response to this question from the chapter: "Has it ever appeared to you, as it did to the first followers, that God just died?"

_____

_____

_____

_____

_____

_____

_____

_____

_____

> JESUS' WORDS—THEN AND NOW—CAN OFFEND.
> THIS IS PRIMARILY BECAUSE, IN EVERY AGE, JESUS IS MORE
> CONCERNED WITH TRUTH THAN DIPLOMACY. HE IS MORE
> DEVOTED TO REALITY THAN TO ILLUSIONS OF PEACE.

Chapter 16

• • •

GROWING PAINS

REFLECT

1. Write out the first of nine encouragements for those who are disillusioned with God:
   When disillusioned with God . . .

   _____

   _____

   _____

   _____

2. "Sometimes we spin our stories to relieve our theological angst. But making excuses for
   God cannot create intimacy with God" (page 83). Think of the generation(s) coming up
   behind you. Have you given them permission to ask angst-filled questions?

   _____

   _____

   _____

   _____

3. If not, why?

   _____

   _____

   _____

   _____

4. "I don't know" is a smart answer when it's true. Many questioners need to be heard even
   more than they need to find answers. Bring to mind the questioners in your life who
   simply need to feel heard.

STUDY

Read 2 Peter 3:17b-18:

> Be on your guard so that you may not be carried away by the error of lawless men and fall from your secure position. But grow in the grace and knowledge of our Lord and Savior Jesus Christ. To him be glory both now and forever! Amen.

1. Peter appears to be contrasting *falling* with *growing* and *error* with *grace*. Though at some point all stop growing physically, what can happen when we stop growing spiritually?

   _____

   _____

   _____

2. Alicia states, "Growth, for all its positives, is still a form of pressure. By definition, growth requires change" (page 81). Share any stories from your own journey that illustrate this principle.

   _____

   _____

   _____

RESPOND

Recount the story of Alicia's friend who had prided herself in never questioning God. (See pages 82–83.) Spend a minute in undistracted silence asking God if there are any questions you need to have the courage to ask Him.

_____

_____

_____

_____

OUR FUTURES WILL BE FORGED MORE BY WHAT WE DO
WITH PAIN THAN BY WHAT WE DO WITH JOY.

Chapter 17

• • •

COOKIES AND CANDOR

REFLECT

1. Write out encouragement 2: When disillusioned with God . . .

_____

_____

_____

2. Starting on page 86, list the scriptural examples offered of disillusionment with God.

_____

_____

_____

_____

3. Recount Alicia's advice to her daughter after the car accident. (See page 88.)

_____

_____

_____

4. How at liberty are you to live sad *with Jesus*?

_____

_____

_____

_____

STUDY

Read John 11:20-23, 32-37:

When Martha heard that Jesus was coming, she went out to meet him, but Mary stayed at home. "Lord," Martha said to Jesus, "if you had been here, my brother would not have died. But I know that even now God will give you whatever you ask." Jesus said to her, "Your brother will rise again." . . . When Mary reached the place where Jesus was and saw him, she fell at his feet and said, "Lord, if you had been here, my brother would not have died." When Jesus saw her weeping, and the Jews who had come along with her also weeping, he was deeply moved in spirit and troubled. "Where have you laid him?" he asked. "Come and see, Lord," they replied. Jesus wept. Then the Jews said, "See how he loved him!" But some of them said, "Could not he who opened the eyes of the blind man have kept this man from dying?"

1. Circle each character and underline each verb in the story.

2. In your own words, what accusation was being made about Jesus in the final sentence?

_____

_____

_____

RESPOND

1. What explanations have you heard about why Jesus wept?

_____

_____

_____

2. Do you believe that Jesus weeps with you? Why or why not?

_____

_____

_____

OUR NIGHTS ADD DEPTH TO OUR DAYS.

Chapter 18

. . .

WHAT DOTS ARE NOT

REFLECT

1. Write out encouragement 3: When disillusioned with God . . .

_____

_____

_____

_____

2. What did Oswald Chambers identify as the danger of theological training?

_____

_____

_____

_____

3. What solution did he offer to this problem? (See pages 91–92.)

_____

_____

_____

_____

CONNECTING DOTS CALMS ME.
BUT I DARE NOT MISTAKE THE CALM FOR FAITH.
FAITH IS RELATIONAL.

STUDY

Read John 20:24-29:

> Now Thomas (called Didymus), one of the Twelve, was not with the disciples when Jesus came. So the other disciples told him, "We have seen the Lord!" But he said to them, "Unless I see the nail marks in his hands and put my finger where the nails were, and put my hand into his side, I will not believe it." A week later his disciples were in the house again, and Thomas was with them. Though the doors were locked, Jesus came and stood among them and said, "Peace be with you!" Then he said to Thomas, "Put your finger here; see my hands. Reach out your hand and put it into my side. Stop doubting and believe." Thomas said to him, "My Lord and my God!" Then Jesus told him, "Because you have seen me, you have believed; blessed are those who have not seen and yet have believed."

1. What specific physical proof did Thomas want before believing that Jesus had risen from the dead?

   _____

   _____

   _____

   _____

2. What would this proof verify?

   _____

   _____

   _____

   _____

3. In mercy, Jesus connected these dots for Thomas. But what did He say about those who believed before that indisputable evidence was tangible?

   _____

   _____

   _____

   _____

RESPOND

1. "We simply cannot think our way out of disillusionment, but we can give our trust-muscles a good workout by choosing to have more confidence in *who God is* than in our ability to connect all the dots" (page 92). Are there any areas in which you tend to place your trust in connecting the dots?

    _____

    _____

    _____

    _____

    _____

2. If so, take a big breath in and with your exhale say, "Lord, I trust you more than I trust myself." Lay down your dot-connecting pen and give your mind a rest.

    _____

    _____

    _____

    _____

    _____

    _____

    _____

    _____

> GOD GAVE US BRAINS. CLEARLY, HE DELIGHTS IN OUR
> USE OF THEM. BUT THINKING IS NOT THE SAME AS TRUSTING.
> AND TRUST—WITH OR WITHOUT UNDERSTANDING—
> IS HOW WE FOLLOW GOD THROUGH THE NIGHT.

Disillusionment with God

For the word of God is living and active. Sharper than any double-edged sword,
it penetrates even to dividing soul and spirit, joints and marrow;
it judges the thoughts and attitudes of the heart.

HEBREWS 4:12

Though he slay me, yet will I hope in him.

JOB 13:15

Chapter 19

· · ·

THIRSTY THOUGHTS

REFLECT

1. Write out encouragement 4: When disillusioned with God . . .

   _____

   _____

   _____

2. Like Alicia, have you ever felt hypocritical reading the Bible when you were disillusioned with God? (See page 94.)

   _____

   _____

   _____

   _____

   _____

3. Look up the definition of *hypocrisy* and then discuss or reflect on the following: "Because the Word is living, continuing to expose ourselves to it when we feel nothing (and believe even less) is not hypocrisy; it is faith" (page 94).

   _____

   _____

   _____

   _____

   _____

STUDY

Read Matthew 4:1-10:

Then Jesus was led by the Spirit into the desert to be tempted by the devil. After fasting forty days and forty nights, he was hungry. The tempter came to him and said, "If you are the Son of God, tell these stones to become bread." Jesus answered, "It is written: 'Man does not live on bread alone, but on every word that comes from the mouth of God.'" Then the devil took him to the holy city and had him stand on the highest point of the temple. "If you are the Son of God," he said, "throw yourself down. For it is written: 'He will command his angels concerning you, and they will lift you up in their hands, so that you will not strike your foot against a stone.'" Jesus answered him, "It is also written: 'Do not put the Lord your God to the test.'" Again, the devil took him to a very high mountain and showed him all the kingdoms of the world and their splendor. "All this I will give you," he said, "if you will bow down and worship me." Jesus said to him, "Away from me, Satan! For it is written: 'Worship the Lord your God, and serve him only.'"

1. In this passage, circle every occurrence of "if" and underline each occurrence of "it is written."

2. Which Scripture verses did Satan quote in the temptation?

3. What can you learn from this passage about Satan's strategies?

4. Describe Jesus' strategy to stay faithful to His Father in the midst of temptation.

RESPOND

"So keep reading and studying the Bible. Keep praying and memorizing the Word. Not because you feel like it, but because within His Voice is the strength you truly need to navigate the night" (page 96).

1. Write out a prayer asking God to strengthen your relationship with His Word. Be sure to include a request for mentors and teachers if you feel you need more tools to grow in this area.

_____

_____

_____

_____

_____

_____

2. Then pause to consider what you can do to partner with God in answer to this prayer.

_____

_____

_____

_____

_____

_____

CHOOSING TO SATURATE OUR THOUGHTS WITH THE SCRIPTURES WHEN WE ARE DISILLUSIONED IS EVIDENCE THAT OUR FAITH IS BASED ON *WHAT IS TRUE*, NOT *WHAT IS FELT*.

Chapter 20

. . .

BODY BUILDING

REFLECT

1. Write out encouragement 5: When disillusioned with God . . .

   _____

   _____

2. In your nights, with regard to your health, what practices have you found to be helpful?

   _____

   _____

   _____

   _____

3. What practices have you found to be hurtful?

   _____

   _____

   _____

   _____

4. "In the night, many speed up, others slow down, and a few, like Elijah, do a bit of both: they run fast and then crash hard" (page 98). Which (if any) pattern do you identify with most closely?

   _____

   _____

   _____

STUDY

Read 3 John 1:2:

> Dear friend, I pray that you may enjoy good health and that all may go well with you, even as your soul is getting along well.

1. What three things does John pray over his friend?

   _____

   _____

2. Rewrite this prayer in your own words and take a few minutes to pray it over a dear friend.

   _____

   _____

   _____

RESPOND

1. Reflect on Elijah's experience of disillusionment. (See chapter 20.) Summarize the God-led steps Elijah took to journey from spiritual exhaustion to spiritual insight.

   _____

   _____

   _____

2. Then ask the Holy Spirit to highlight any steps you need to incorporate into this season of your life.

   _____

   _____

   _____

SOMETIMES OUR HEALTH CAN TAKE A HIT IN THE NIGHT
NOT BECAUSE OF THE DARKNESS,
BUT FROM THE FALLOUT OF OUR COPING MECHANISMS.

Chapter 21

. . .

IN THE MOURNING

REFLECT

1. Write out encouragement 6: When disillusioned with God . . .

_____

_____

_____

2. Reread the list of graveside doubts from page 101. Are there any others from your personal experience that you can add?

_____

_____

_____

_____

_____

_____

_____

_____

_____

_____

STUDY

Read Luke 23:49–24:16, excerpts of which are below.

Going to Pilate, [Joseph] asked for Jesus' body. Then he took it down, wrapped it in linen cloth and placed it in a tomb cut in the rock, one in which no one had yet been laid. (23:52-53)

The women who had come with Jesus from Galilee followed Joseph and saw the tomb and how his body was laid in it. Then they went home and prepared spices and perfumes. But they rested on the Sabbath in obedience to the commandment. On the first day of the week, very early in the morning, the women took the spices they had prepared and went to the tomb. (23:55–24:1)

When they came back from the tomb, they told all these things to the Eleven and to all the others. (24:9)

Peter, however, got up and ran to the tomb. Bending over, he saw the strips of linen lying by themselves, and he went away, wondering to himself what had happened. Now that same day two of them were going to a village called Emmaus, about seven miles from Jerusalem. They were talking with each other about everything that had happened. As they talked and discussed these things with each other, Jesus himself came up and walked along with them; but they were kept from recognizing him. (24:12-16)

1. Circle every verb in these verses. Then underline each word or phrase that shows what the disciples of Jesus *did* after His crucifixion.

2. If you were writing this chapter in *The Night Is Normal*, what words would you have chosen to describe how the disciples processed the death of the greatest dream they had ever known?

_____

_____

_____

_____

_____

_____

_____

_____

_____

_____

_____

_____

RESPOND

"Like the disciples, we need time to process loss when we are disillusioned. . . . Take the time, my friend. Prepare the spices. Preserve and honor the memories" (page 102).

Find a quiet place and take a few deep breaths with Jesus. Give yourself permission to grieve safely in His presence.

> MOVING THROUGH DISILLUSIONMENT TOWARD LOVE DOES NOT MEAN THAT WE DO NOT GRIEVE, BUT RATHER, THAT WE PROCESS OUR SORROW SINCERELY WITH OUR SAVIOR.

Chapter 22

. . .

PROOF MISUSE

REFLECT

1. Write out encouragement 7: When disillusioned with God . . .

_____

_____

_____

2. "If-thens are dangerous because they masquerade as truth. And untruth, if not identified and evaluated, has the power to undo belief" (page 105). Consider those who no longer believe in Jesus. What untruths may have contributed to their departure from the faith?

_____

_____

_____

_____

_____

3. Reread the if-thens listed on page 106. Thinking of a parent-child relationship, what childhood if-thens are often shattered by healthy parenting?

_____

_____

_____

_____

_____

STUDY

Read Psalm 37:1-9:

> Do not fret because of evil men or be envious of those who do wrong; for like the grass they will soon wither, like green plants they will soon die away. Trust in the LORD and do good; dwell in the land and enjoy safe pasture. Delight yourself in the LORD and he will give you the desires of your heart. Commit your way to the LORD; trust in him and he will do this: He will make your righteousness shine like the dawn, the justice of your cause like the noonday sun. Be still before the LORD and wait patiently for him; do not fret when men succeed in their ways, when they carry out their wicked schemes. Refrain from anger and turn from wrath; do not fret—it leads only to evil. For evil men will be cut off, but those who hope in the LORD will inherit the land.

1. On one side of the column below, list what this passage tells us to do. On the other side, list what this passage states that God will do.

WHAT GOD CALLS US TO DO	WHAT GOD WILL DO

2. Which side do you most often focus upon?

_____

_____

_____

3. Slowly read aloud each line in this chapter's closing prayer.

RESPOND

1. Respond to the following as honestly as possible.

   If I serve God with all my might, then _____.

   If God really loves me, then _____.

2. Ask God to edit any unhealthy equations that are shaping your soul as you whisper Job's declaration: "Though he slay me, yet will I hope in him" (Job 13:15).

   _____

   _____

   _____

   _____

   _____

   _____

   _____

   _____

   _____

   _____

   _____

THOUGH WE AGREE THAT REDUCING FAITH TO A FORMULA IS ABSURD, EQUATIONS STILL SNEAK THEIR WAY INTO OUR BELIEF SYSTEMS. THEY FORM IN THE SHADOWS OF OUR ASSUMPTIONS AND ARE EXPOSED—NOT BY DAY, BUT BY NIGHT.

Chapter 23

. . .

A LIFELINE

REFLECT

1. Write out encouragement 8: When disillusioned with God . . .

_____

_____

_____

_____

2. Share any stories of your Josettes (see pages 111–113), of those who gave to you in the midst of their own pain.

_____

_____

_____

_____

_____

_____

_____

_____

> WHEN WE ARE DISILLUSIONED, ACTIVATING EVEN
> A LITTLE BIT OF COMPASSION CAN SERVE TO GUARD
> OUR EMOTIONAL AND MENTAL WELL-BEING.

STUDY

Read Isaiah 53:3:

> He was despised and rejected by men, a man of sorrows, and familiar with suffering. Like one from whom men hide their faces he was despised, and we esteemed him not.

1. Underline any descriptions of the Messiah that you believe are *past tense* with one line and any that you believe are *present tense* with two lines.

2. Discuss how you made your decisions.

_____

_____

_____

_____

_____

RESPOND

Recall the illustration of a waterwheel on pages 110–111. Below, write out a declaration personalizing Alicia's encouragement to "refuse to let disillusionment pass by without activating something within [you] to help others" (page 111).

_____

_____

_____

_____

_____

_____

IS THE GOSPEL SIMPLE? PERHAPS. BUT GOD HAS NEVER BEEN AND WILL NEVER BE SIMPLISTIC. GOD NEVER DILUTES DISCREPANCY NOR IGNORES COMPLEXITY. HE DOES NOT CONVENIENTLY EDIT OUT THE UNCOMFORTABLE. GOD IS THE ULTIMATE REALIST. HE IS NO STRANGER TO PAIN.

Chapter 24

. . .

THE UNGLAMOROUS
GIFT

REFLECT

1. Write out encouragement 9: When disillusioned with God . . .

_____

_____

2. What does Alicia mean by "plod on"?

_____

_____

3. List the challenges William Carey plodded through. (See pages 116–117.)

_____

_____

_____

_____

4. How might you have felt toward God if you lived Carey's life?

_____

_____

_____

_____

_____

STUDY

Read Luke 9:51:

> As the time approached for him to be taken up to heaven, Jesus resolutely set out for Jerusalem.

1. What is the definition of *resolutely?*

   _____

   _____

2. Knowing what awaited Him, how do you think Jesus found the strength to plod on?

   _____

   _____

3. Can any of His motivations still strengthen you today?

   _____

   _____

   _____

   _____

RESPOND

Reread the examples offered of those who plodded on (see page 117). Then add to that list the names of holy plodders you have personally observed or known.

_____

_____

_____

_____

SPIRITUALLY, *PLODDING* IS ABOUT MOVING FORWARD,
NOT BY LEAPS AND BOUNDS OVER TALL BUILDINGS, BUT BY
CHOICES AND TEARS THROUGH PAIN-FILLED NIGHTS.

Chapter 25

· · ·

ON THE OTHER SIDE

REFLECT

1. In telling the rest of the story about Rachel, Alicia states: "Grief did not lead her to bail; bitterness did" (page 121). How would you describe the difference between grief and bitterness?

_____

_____

_____

2. Alicia speaks of a difference in the lives of those who choose the way of love in the midst of pain as "a scent of heaven mingling with the tears of earth; a richness of character that can neither be feigned nor fabricated" (page 122). Who comes to mind when you think of a soul that exemplifies such richness?

_____

_____

_____

STUDY

Read Joshua 24:14-15:

Now fear the LORD and serve him with all faithfulness. Throw away the gods your forefathers worshiped beyond the River and in Egypt, and serve the LORD. But if serving the LORD seems undesirable to you, then choose for yourselves this day whom you will serve, whether the gods your forefathers served beyond the River, or the gods of the Amorites, in whose land you are living. But as for me and my household, we will serve the LORD.

Discuss the context of this often-quoted verse in light of the following quote: "My friend, never underestimate what or who is awaiting you on the other side of your disillusionment. More depends on your choice to keep loving God than you can imagine. The destiny of nations could rest on the choices you make today in the depth of the night" (page 122).

_____

_____

_____

_____

_____

_____

RESPOND

1. Craft a sentence listing the pains you are currently navigating, but end the sentence with a comma, not a period.

_____

_____

_____

_____

_____

_____

2. Then reread John 6:68 and add, "but to whom shall I go, Lord, but to you."

_____

_____

YOU AND YOUR FAITH ARE IRREPLACEABLE.
YOUR COMMITMENT TO FOLLOW JESUS, ESPECIALLY
THROUGH THE NIGHT, IS A POWERFUL WEAPON
AGAINST THE FORCES OF EVIL ON THIS EARTH.

• • •

Disillusionment
with Self

As a father has compassion on his children, so the LORD has compassion on those who fear him; for he knows how we are formed, he remembers that we are dust.

PSALM 103:13–14

Chapter 26

. . .

SPIRITUAL FRUSTRATION

REFLECT

1. What does it mean to spiritually be disillusioned with your self? (See page 127.)

_____

_____

_____

_____

2. What is the link between frustration and deception? (See page 128.)

_____

_____

_____

_____

3. Reflecting on Psalm 103:14 in the context of being disillusioned with self, Alicia asserts that "Seeing ourselves as dust, however, can be painful. Committing to God in the midst of that pain will require us to value His presence more than our quantifiable progress" (page 129). Rephrase this principle in your own words.

_____

_____

_____

_____

STUDY

Read Colossians 3:1-3:

> Since, then, you have been raised with Christ, set your hearts on things above, where Christ is seated at the right hand of God. Set your minds on things above, not on earthly things. For you died, and your life is now hidden with Christ in God.

1. Underline *what* Paul admonished the Colossians to do. Then circle or highlight the *why*.

2. In your own words, how is the *why* a sufficient motivation for the *what*?

_____

_____

_____

_____

3. What does "set" mean in the phrases "set your hearts" and "set your minds"?

_____

_____

4. Have you ever successfully trained a puppy to *sit*? If so, describe that process. For example, what steps did you take? What obstacles did you and the puppy have to overcome?

_____

_____

_____

_____

_____

5. How successfully do you feel you've trained yourself to *set* your mind and heart on things above?

_____

_____

_____

_____

6. How can the puppy-training example encourage and instruct you?

_____

_____

_____

_____

RESPOND

1. Respond to Alicia's question: "Have you ever felt let down by what you thought were reasonable, Bible-based expectations?" (page 128).

_____

_____

_____

_____

_____

2. If so, talk with God honestly about those frustrations. Begin with "God, when Your Word said _____, I thought for sure that meant _____."

_____

_____

_____

_____

_____

_____

> BEING NEW IS A GIVEN FOR THOSE WHO BELIEVE.
> HOWEVER, WALKING OUT THAT NEWNESS ALMOST ALWAYS
> INITIATES DISILLUSIONMENT ABOUT OUR
> HUMANITY, IN GENERAL, AND OUR FAITH, IN PARTICULAR.

Chapter 27

. . .

SOMETHING OLD

REFLECT

1. Recount Alicia's story of personal disillusionment when her fifth-year cancer scan did not confirm her interpretation of the peace she had been experiencing.

_____

_____

_____

2. Discuss any way in which Alicia's conclusion feels familiar: "I had peace because I had Jesus. He was with me and was leading me . . . straight into a desert" (page 132).

_____

_____

_____

_____

STUDY

Read Psalm 42:5, 11:

Why are you downcast, O my soul? Why so disturbed within me? Put your hope in God, for I will yet praise him, my Savior and my God.

1. Paraphrase this repeated sentence in your own words.

_____

_____

_____

2. "I *know* what's true! Why isn't that changing how I *feel*?" (page 130). Is this frustration familiar to your generation?

_____

_____

_____

_____

_____

_____

RESPOND

Recall the illustration Alicia offers of the small, berm-encircled pool. (See page 133.) Ask God if there's any way in which you, too, have been "trying to tame and contain your grief" with your logic.

_____

_____

_____

_____

_____

_____

> I WEPT—AND HAVE, ON OCCASION, KEPT WEEPING—WITH
> CONFIDENCE THAT MY TEARS (AND NOT JUST MY MIND) HAVE
> AN ASSIGNMENT IN THE MIDST OF SPIRITUAL PAIN.

Chapter 28

. . .

SOMETHING NEW

REFLECT

1. Alicia states that "Getting things wrong is part of growing faith up" (page 136). We understand that mistakes are teachers when we are learning a skill or a sport. Why do you think it's more difficult to accept mistakes as part of the learning process when it comes to learning to follow Jesus?

2. What is gained when you lose illusions about yourself? (See page 136.)

STUDY

Read Matthew 16:16-23:

Simon Peter answered, "You are the Christ, the Son of the living God." Jesus replied, "Blessed are you, Simon son of Jonah, for this was not revealed to you by man, but by my Father in heaven. And I tell you that you are Peter, and on this rock I will build my church, and the gates of Hades will not overcome it. I will give you the keys of the kingdom of heaven; whatever you bind on earth will be bound in heaven, and whatever you loose on earth will be loosed in heaven." Then he warned his disciples not to tell anyone that he was the Christ. From that time on Jesus began to explain to his disciples that he must go to Jerusalem and suffer many things at the hands of the elders, chief priests and teachers of the law, and that he must be killed and on the third day be raised to life. Peter took him aside and began to rebuke him. "Never, Lord!" he said. "This shall never happen to you!" Jesus turned and said to Peter, "Get behind me, Satan! You are a stumbling block to me; you do not have in mind the things of God, but the things of men."

1. To keep this familiar passage fresh in your heart, underline each positive statement Jesus spoke to Peter. Now see yourself as Peter in the story, listening to these words in the presence of the other disciples.

2. Next picture yourself rebuking Jesus for what you perceive as negativity and hear Jesus' response.

3. How might Peter have felt when Jesus rebuked him?

4. What thoughts might he have had about Jesus? About himself?

RESPOND

1. When was the last time you were disillusioned with yourself?

_____
_____
_____
_____
_____
_____
_____

2. What feelings and thoughts did you have during that time?

_____
_____
_____
_____
_____
_____
_____
_____

WHEN AN EARTHQUAKE REVEALS
INTERNAL FAULT LINES THAT YOU NEVER KNEW EXISTED—
WHEN THE GROUND SHAKES BENEATH YOUR FEET
AND YOU FALL INTO DISILLUSIONMENT WITH YOURSELF—
REMEMBER TO GET BACK UP, RECEIVE FORGIVENESS,
AND CALL UPON YOUR NEWLY ACQUIRED HUMILITY
TO INSPIRE OTHERS TO COMMIT TO THE WAY OF LOVE.

Chapter 29

. . .

CHASING HORSES

REFLECT

1. Write out the first of eight encouragements in this section: When disillusioned with yourself . . .

   _____

   _____

2. When you are spiritually disappointed with yourself, where do your thoughts tend to wander?

   _____

   _____

3. What difference might it make in such seasons if you passed your self-talk through the filter Alicia suggests of "Jesus, do _we_ want to think about this right now?" (page 140).

   _____

   _____

STUDY

Read Philippians 4:8:

Finally, brothers, whatever is true, whatever is noble, whatever is right, whatever is pure, whatever is lovely, whatever is admirable—if anything is excellent or praiseworthy—think about such things.

1. Imagine yourself as Peter once again, but this time right after he had denied knowledge of Jesus three times and the rooster had crowed. Brainstorm self-talk applications from Philippians 4:8 for Peter's situation. For example,

Whatever is true →
Jesus knew this would happen. It didn't surprise Him.

Whatever is noble →

_____

Whatever is right →

_____

Whatever is pure →

_____

Whatever is lovely →

_____

Whatever is admirable →

_____

Anything that is excellent or praiseworthy →

_____

2. How can thinking *with* God, instead of just *about* God, help us be faithful to Paul's admonition?

_____

_____

RESPOND

How might asking God to mentor your mind affect your self-talk in disillusioning times?

_____

_____

_____

INSTEAD OF "DO *I* WANT TO THINK ABOUT THIS RIGHT NOW?"
ASK, "JESUS, DO *WE* WANT TO THINK ABOUT THIS RIGHT NOW?"

Chapter 30

. . .

HEART MATTERS

REFLECT

1. Write out encouragement 2: When disillusioned with yourself . . .

   _____

   _____

2. Job's friends spoke passionately but in error. What premise were they operating from that made their counsel "miserable" (Job 16:2)? (See page 144.)

   _____

   _____

3. Recount the four biblical signs of spiritual growth from Alicia's teaching on pages 145–146. (Be sure to consult this chapter's endnotes for the Scripture references.)

   _____

   _____

   _____

   _____

STUDY

Read Hebrews 11:32-39:

And what more shall I say? I do not have time to tell about Gideon, Barak, Samson, Jephthah, David, Samuel and the prophets, who through faith conquered kingdoms, administered justice, and gained what was promised; who shut the mouths of lions, quenched the fury of the flames, and escaped the edge of the sword; whose weakness was turned to strength; and who became powerful in battle and routed foreign armies.

Women received back their dead, raised to life again. Others were tortured and refused to be released, so that they might gain a better resurrection. Some faced jeers and flogging, while still others were chained and put in prison. They were stoned; they were sawed in two; they were put to death by the sword. They went about in sheepskins and goatskins, destitute, persecuted and mistreated—the world was not worthy of them. They wandered in deserts and mountains, and in caves and holes in the ground. These were all commended for their faith.

1. Consider this quote from page 144: "Especially if we have known privilege, we must be vigilant to avoid confusing abundance for obedience or social success for the favor of God." Draw a line through the verses the author of Hebrews might have omitted if he had suffered from this confusion, if he had mistaken prosperity for devotion.

2. Reflecting on the four biblical signs of spiritual growth from pages 145–146, in what ways do you see that your faith is growing?

RESPOND

As you've read through this chapter, were you able to identify any signs of growth you were looking for in yourself that weren't biblical or spiritual? If so, write them below.

EVIDENTLY, PROSPERITY, EASE, STABILITY, SUCCESS, AND RELIGIOUS SPEECH ARE NOT ABSOLUTE INDICATORS OF SPIRITUAL GROWTH. SPIRITUAL GROWTH IS A MATTER OF THE HEART.

Chapter 31

. . .

THAT SAME OLD SPOT

REFLECT

1. Write out encouragement 3: When disillusioned with yourself . . .

_____

_____

2. Have you ever felt discouraged about your spiritual growth? If so, are any of the thoughts Alicia lists at the bottom of page 148 familiar?

_____

_____

_____

_____

_____

_____

3. How might thinking of spiritual growth as more of a spiral than a straight line affect your self-perception?

_____

_____

_____

_____

_____

4. Your interaction with others?

_____

_____

_____

_____

STUDY

Read 2 Corinthians 3:17-18:

Now the Lord is the Spirit, and where the Spirit of the Lord is, there is freedom. And we, who with unveiled faces all reflect the Lord's glory, are being transformed into his likeness with ever-increasing glory, which comes from the Lord, who is the Spirit.

1. In this verse, "are being transformed into" is translated from the Greek word *metamorphoumetha*. In a dictionary, look up the words *transform* and *metamorphosis*, and write the definitions below.

_____

_____

_____

2. Personalize and reiterate this verse with your own words. For example, "I, [*insert your name here*], reflect God's glory . . ."

_____

_____

_____

_____

_____

> FORGIVENESS IS DEPENDENT UPON JESUS' SACRIFICIAL OFFERING, NOT OUR PERFECT ASKING. SINCERE REPENTANCE IS MOST CERTAINLY HEARD BY THE GOD WHO KNOWS AND LOVES US FULLY.

RESPOND

1. Personally, has most of your spiritual growth felt like Alicia's surgery or her dad's? (See pages 149–150.)

_____

_____

_____

_____

_____

_____

_____

2. Ask God to strengthen your hope in the longer surgeries in your life.

_____

_____

_____

_____

_____

_____

_____

ADDRESSING AN OLD ISSUE IN A NEW SEASON IS
OFTEN A SIGN OF GROWTH, NOT OF FAILURE.

• • •

Disillusionment with Self

WEEK 6, CHAPTERS 32–37

To keep me from becoming conceited because of these surpassingly great revelations, there was given me a thorn in my flesh, a messenger of Satan, to torment me. Three times I pleaded with the Lord to take it away from me. But he said to me, "My grace is sufficient for you, for my power is made perfect in weakness." Therefore I will boast all the more gladly about my weaknesses, so that Christ's power may rest on me.

2 CORINTHIANS 12:7-9

Chapter 32

. . .

GAINING GROUND

REFLECT

1. Write out encouragement 4: When disillusioned with yourself . . .

_____

_____

_____

2. Recalling the story of the man who struggled with impurity, reflect on this quote: "Defining a word as weighty as _victory_ through the presence or absence of something as flighty as feelings will continually place victory out of our reach" (page 154).

_____

_____

_____

3. How common do you think it is for Christians to wait for their feelings to change before declaring victory in their lives? (See pages 153–154.)

_____

_____

_____

_____

_____

_____

_____

4. Alicia points out that in the Garden of Gethsemane, Jesus' feelings weren't in sync with His Father's will, yet He neither sinned nor failed. (See pages 155–156.) How could Jesus be victorious when His emotions were uncooperative?

_____

_____

_____

_____

_____

_____

_____

VICTORY SOURCED IN FEELINGS IS NOT VIABLE.

STUDY

Read Romans 7:18-23:

I know that nothing good lives in me, that is, in my sinful nature. For I have the desire to do what is good, but I cannot carry it out. For what I do is not the good I want to do; no, the evil I do not want to do—this I keep on doing. Now if I do what I do not want to do, it is no longer I who do it, but it is sin living in me that does it. So I find this law at work: When I want to do good, evil is right there with me. For in my inner being I delight in God's law; but I see another law at work in the members of my body, waging war against the law of my mind and making me a prisoner of the law of sin at work within my members.

1. In this passage, underline with one line the good Paul wants to do and with two lines what he actually found himself doing.

NOT ONLY IS VICTORY THE STUFF OF CHOICES
(NOT FEELINGS), VICTORY CAN BE VALIDLY CELEBRATED
EACH "INSTANCE OR OCCASION" OF ACTION,
NOT JUST AFTER THE ENTIRE WAR HAS BEEN WON.

2. "Just do it!" is a popular mantra. In your own words, what factors weighed down Paul's will to "just do" good?

_____

_____

_____

3. Are any of these forces familiar to you?

_____

_____

_____

_____

_____

RESPOND

Ask God to reveal to you any area in which you have thrown in the towel of defeat too soon, any area in which you have mistaken the absence of cooperative emotions for the absence of victory.

_____

_____

_____

_____

_____

_____

OUR GENERATION IS BEING HELD BACK BY THE FALLACY
THAT *DOING* SOMETHING WITHOUT FIRST *FEELING* SOMETHING
IS HYPOCRITICAL. LIKE JOE, WE SIT DISILLUSIONED
WITH OURSELVES NEEDLESSLY, WAITING FOR OUR FEELINGS
TO CHANGE IN ORDER FOR US TO DECLARE VICTORY.

Chapter 33

. . .

NEVER WASTED

REFLECT

1. Write out encouragement 5: When disillusioned with yourself . . .

2. Share ways in which God has guided you into His will through weakness.

3. Retell the lesson Alicia learned from the splinters. (See pages 159–160.)

GOD DOES NOT SHOW US OUR WEAKNESS TO MOCK US.
GOD REVEALS TO HEAL.

STUDY

Read Philippians 1:3-6:

> I thank my God every time I remember you. In all my prayers for all of you, I always pray with joy because of your partnership in the gospel from the first day until now, being confident of this, that he who began a good work in you will carry it on to completion until the day of Christ Jesus.

Will carry it on to completion is translated from the Greek *epitelesei* (to accomplish, to bring about, to complete), which also appears in 2 Corinthians 8:6, 11. What do you think Paul meant by "*epitelesei* until the day of Christ Jesus"?

RESPOND

Spend time in prayer responding to Alicia's final encouragement in this chapter: "When disillusioned with ourselves, let us lean in to listen for God's whispers, knowing that somehow, His 'power is made perfect in [our] weakness' (2 Corinthians 12:9)."

WHEN ELIJAH FELT LIKE A FAILURE AND WAS DISILLUSIONED
WITH HIMSELF TO THE POINT OF DESPAIR, GOD CAME TO
HIM—NOT IN THE POWER OF WIND, EARTHQUAKE, OR FIRE,
BUT IN A GENTLE WHISPER. GOD STILL WHISPERS TO US
IN OUR WEAKNESS. WISDOM INVITES US TO LISTEN.

Chapter 34

. . .

FILTERING "FAILURES"

REFLECT

1. Write out encouragement 6: When disillusioned with yourself . . .

   _____

   _____

   _____

2. Alicia states, "Did Jesus die on the cross *to forgive me* for holding an evangelistic aerobics outreach? No. Not at all. *Because not all failure is sin*" (page 162). Share any thoughts or feelings you had while reading Alicia's story and conclusion.

   _____

   _____

   _____

   _____

   _____

3. If you had been her campus pastor, do you think you would have given her the green light to pursue an idea you felt would fail? Why or why not?

   _____

   _____

   _____

   _____

   _____

4. Underline the responses that are most common when you or your peers are processing personal failure.

Don't think about it.

Personalize the failure. (*Then I'm a failure too.*)

Move on to whatever is next.

Go faster to outrun the discomfort.

Beat yourself up about it.

Refuse to forgive yourself.

Rationalize it.

Become depressed.

Go to God.

Tell others.

Try to make up for it elsewhere.

Sin more.

Deny that there was a failure. (*Everything's fine.*)

Eat chocolate.

5. Discuss the four possibilities this chapter identifies when you're faced with a perceived spiritual failure. (See pages 164–165.)

_____

_____

_____

_____

> HOW WE DEFINE FAILURE MATTERS BECAUSE
> WHAT WE SAY TO OURSELVES WHEN DISILLUSIONED IS FORMATIVE.
> ACCURACY STRENGTHENS US. INACCURACY DOES NOT.

STUDY

Read Luke 22:31-34:

"Simon, Simon, Satan has asked to sift you as wheat. But I have prayed for you, Simon, that your faith may not fail. And when you have turned back, strengthen your brothers." But he replied, "Lord, I am ready to go with you to prison and to death." Jesus answered, "I tell you, Peter, before the rooster crows today, you will deny three times that you know me."

1. What did Jesus know about Peter that Peter did not yet know about himself?

_____

_____

_____

2. What future hope did Jesus offer Peter in this revelation?

_____

_____

3. Peter did deny Jesus. And Peter did "turn back" and fulfill Jesus' request to "strengthen [his] brothers." Do you believe that Peter's faith failed?

_____

_____

RESPOND

1. How often do you call yourself a failure in your self-talk?

_____

_____

_____

2. How might that frequency be affected if you first filtered your accusation through the three questions Alicia offers?

   Did Jesus die for this?
   Did I do this in disobedience?
   Did I numb myself to or simply ignore the conviction of the Spirit? (page 164).

_____

_____

_____

_____

_____

_____

_____

_____

_____

NOT ALL FAILURE IS SIN. IN FACT, FAILURE IS ONE OF THE WISEST
TEACHERS IN THE GROWTH PROCESS (IF WE LET IT SPEAK).

Chapter 35

. . .

PICKLE SOUP

REFLECT

1. Write out encouragement 7: When disillusioned with yourself . . .

   _____

   _____

2. In your own words, what are Alicia's concerns about some of the ways in which our art has historically shaped our view of Jesus? (See pages 166–167.)

   _____

   _____

3. Brainstorm responses to Alicia's question: "Surely baby Jesus bawled. Crying is not a sin. And surely Jesus looked like an agonized mess in Gethsemane the night He was betrayed. Feeling sorrowful is not a sin. Why then do our depictions sometimes tidy Him up?" (page 167).

   _____

   _____

   _____

4. Together, process the following four questions Alicia asks on pages 167–168.

   Imagine baby Jesus taking His first step. Do you see Him teetering and falling or standing the first time (and being selected for the Olympics shortly afterward)?

   _____

   _____

   _____

Imagine Jesus attending a school that may have been connected to the local synagogue. Do you think He had the highest grades in the class? Is it conceivable that He might have had something less than an A in math?

_____

_____

Imagine a track team at this hypothetical school. Do you assume that Jesus would have been the fastest? Could someone else have been the captain of the team?

_____

_____

Imagine Jesus crafting a bench in Joseph's shop. Do you think His first work was His best work? Is it possible that He had to scrap it and try again?

_____

_____

5. Why do you think many struggle to distinguish between growth curves and failure?

_____

_____

_____

_____

6. What is the point of the story Alicia shared about her daughter's pickle soup? (See pages 170–171.)

_____

_____

_____

STUDY

Read Luke 2:39-40, 51-52:

When Joseph and Mary had done everything required by the Law of the Lord, they returned to Galilee to their own town of Nazareth. And the child grew and became strong; he was filled with wisdom, and the grace of God was upon him. . . . Then he went down to

Nazareth with them and was obedient to them. But his mother treasured all these things in her heart. And Jesus grew in wisdom and stature, and in favor with God and men.

1. Highlight or underline the ways in which Jesus grew. (See page 169.)

_____

_____

2. Are any of these ways easier for you to understand and/or accept than others? Why?

_____

_____

_____

RESPOND

1. Respond to Alicia's question on page 168: "Do [I] give [myself] permission *to be human and grow?*"

_____

_____

_____

2. Prayerfully discern if you see yourself in these words: "Sometimes we are disillusioned with ourselves not because we are losing illusions and gaining reality (which is healthy), but because we have not given ourselves permission *to be human* (which is unsustainable)" (page 171).

_____

_____

_____

_____

> JESUS *GREW*. GROWING IS NOT FAILURE. GROWING MEANS
> THAT WE ARE MORE TODAY THAN WE WERE YESTERDAY.
> IF THIS WAS TRUE OF JESUS, SURELY IT CAN BE TRUE OF US.

Chapter 36

. . .

THE COMMON THREAD

REFLECT

1. Write out encouragement 8: When disillusioned with yourself . . .

   _____

   _____

2. Why does Alicia believe that an honorable stewardship of God's grace is essential to live out this encouragement? (See pages 173–174.)

   _____

   _____

   _____

   _____

3. How can "an anything-goes religion . . . abuse the gift of grace"? (page 173).

   _____

   _____

   _____

   _____

4. What does and doesn't Alicia mean by the phrase "expecting too much of ourselves"? (See page 173.)

   _____

   _____

   _____

5. Think of the various cultures that have shaped you. Did they lean more toward a view of faith as a performance or as a pilgrimage? In what ways?

_____

_____

_____

_____

_____

_____

_____

6. In what ways can fear turn our faith into more of a performance than a pilgrimage? (See pages 174–175.)

_____

_____

_____

_____

_____

_____

_____

STUDY

Read Isaiah 43:1-5:

But now, this is what the LORD says—he who created you, O Jacob, he who formed you, O Israel: "Fear not, for I have redeemed you; I have summoned you by name; you are mine. When you pass through the waters, I will be with you; and when you pass through the rivers, they will not sweep over you. When you walk through the fire, you will not be burned; the flames will not set you ablaze. For I am the LORD, your God, the Holy One of Israel, your Savior; I give Egypt for your ransom, Cush and Seba in your stead. Since you are precious and honored in my sight, and because I love you, I will give men in exchange for you, and people in exchange for your life. Do not be afraid, for I am with you; I will bring your children from the east and gather you from the west."

Written to God's disillusioned people in captivity in Babylon, God twice calls them to not fear and then gives them the why. Looking at verses 1 and 5, what was that why? On what basis did God inspire His people to break their alliance with fear?

_____

_____

_____

_____

RESPOND

"If we view faith as a performance, we often see God as a critic, watching our every move with skeptical eyes, red pen in hand, evaluating us by criteria beyond anyone's reach. . . . If we view faith as a pilgrimage, we will see God as our Companion, Guide, and Destination" (page 175). Ask God if there are any ways in which your God-concept needs editing.

_____

_____

_____

_____

_____

_____

_____

_____

_____

WHAT WE FEAR VARIES, BUT FEAR ITSELF IS NOT PICKY.
IT GLADLY BOLTS THROUGH ANY OPEN DOOR
TO STEAL GROUND AWAY FROM LOVE.

Chapter 37

. . .

BREATHE DEEPLY

REFLECT

1. In what ways were Peter's and Judas's journeys similar? (See pages 176–178.)

_____

_____

_____

_____

2. What seems to have accounted for their very different endings?

_____

_____

_____

_____

_____

3. What do you think Alicia meant by the following statements: "Grace is received, not earned. Grace's pardon cannot be purchased *by* us because it has already been paid *for* us. Our role is to accept it. In order to do so, all illusions of self-redemption must be abandoned" (page 177)?

_____

_____

_____

_____

STUDY

Read John 21:1-7:

> Afterward Jesus appeared again to his disciples, by the Sea of Tiberias. It happened this way: Simon Peter, Thomas (called Didymus), Nathanael from Cana in Galilee, the sons of Zebedee, and two other disciples were together. "I'm going out to fish," Simon Peter told them, and they said, "We'll go with you." So they went out and got into the boat, but that night they caught nothing. Early in the morning, Jesus stood on the shore, but the disciples did not realize that it was Jesus. He called out to them, "Friends, haven't you any fish?" "No," they answered. He said, "Throw your net on the right side of the boat and you will find some." When they did, they were unable to haul the net in because of the large number of fish. Then the disciple whom Jesus loved said to Peter, "It is the Lord!" As soon as Simon Peter heard him say, "It is the Lord," he wrapped his outer garment around him (for he had taken it off) and jumped into the water.

1. When Peter realized that it was Jesus, what emotions or thoughts might he have experienced that prompted him to jump into the water and get to Jesus quickly?

_____

_____

2. What choices must he have made to not let shame keep him in the boat?

_____

_____

_____

3. Pause to pray. Ask God if shame is keeping you stuck in any boats instead of doing everything you can to get near to Jesus.

_____

_____

_____

_____

_____

_____

_____

RESPOND

1. Both before and after Peter's epic failure, Jesus wanted Peter near Him. Thoughtfully speak to the Lord, identifying ways in which you are disillusioned with yourself.

_____

_____

_____

_____

_____

_____

2. Then thank Him for faithfully staying near you.

_____

_____

_____

_____

_____

_____

_____

GRACE IS RECEIVED, NOT EARNED. GRACE'S PARDON
CANNOT BE PURCHASED *BY* US BECAUSE IT HAS
ALREADY BEEN PAID *FOR* US.

Disillusionment with Others

WEEK 7, CHAPTERS 38–44

Two are better than one, because they have a good return for their work:
If one falls down, his friend can help him up.
But pity the man who falls and has no one to help him up!

ECCLESIASTES 4:9-10

Chapter 38

. . .

(NOT SO)
WELL WITH MY SOUL

REFLECT

1. Of the three forms of disillusionment discussed in *The Night Is Normal*, which have been the most painful for you to navigate: disillusionment with God, self, or the people of God?

_____

_____

_____

_____

2. Briefly summarize the story of Horatio Spafford. (See pages 183–185.)

_____

_____

_____

_____

3. Have you ever experienced a season in which others judged your pain—as the church once did with the Spaffords—and concluded that you were reaping what you sowed?

_____

_____

_____

_____

_____

_____

4. "When disillusioned with God's people, committing to the upward pull of love not only guides us through the night, it keeps our wounds uninfected along the way" (page 186). What evidence is there that the Spaffords worked to keep their wounds uninfected?

_____

_____

_____

_____

_____

_____

_____

_____

STUDY

Read Philippians 1:12-18:

Now I want you to know, brothers, that what has happened to me has really served to advance the gospel. As a result, it has become clear throughout the whole palace guard and to everyone else that I am in chains for Christ. Because of my chains, most of the brothers in the Lord have been encouraged to speak the word of God more courageously and fearlessly. It is true that some preach Christ out of envy and rivalry, but others out of goodwill. The latter do so in love, knowing that I am put here for the defense of the gospel. The former preach Christ out of selfish ambition, not sincerely, supposing that they can stir up trouble for me while I am in chains. But what does it matter? The important thing is that in every way, whether from false motives or true, Christ is preached. And because of this I rejoice. Yes, and I will continue to rejoice.

1. Underline and then describe the relational pain around God's table that's evident in this passage.

_____

_____

_____

_____

_____

_____

_____

_____

2. How do you think Paul managed to keep rejoicing?

_____

_____

_____

_____

_____

_____

RESPOND

Read Horatio's hymn on page 185 aloud as a prayer. Do any lines especially stand out to you?

_____

_____

_____

_____

_____

_____

_____

_____

MOST OF US, SINCE AROUND KINDERGARTEN, HAVE
UNDERSTOOD THAT THE ONLY WAY TO AVOID PEOPLE PROBLEMS
IS TO AVOID PEOPLE. LIFE TOGETHER GUARANTEES DRAMA.
BUT WHEN PAIN IS SERVED TO US AT GOD'S TABLE,
LET ALONE IN GOD'S NAME, WE CAN ENTER A NIGHT
THAT IS EXTREMELY DIFFICULT TO NEGOTIATE.

Chapter 39

. . .

SOMETHING OLD
AND SOMETHING NEW

REFLECT

1. Review Alicia's list of disillusionment in the family of God from the first book of the Old Testament. (See pages 187–188.)

2. Though anything we offer can only be a guess, why do you think God inspired the author of Genesis to record such embarrassing drama for all the ages?

_____

_____

_____

_____

STUDY

1. Read aloud the New Testament examples of interpersonal disillusionment found on pages 189–190. Then in a word or phrase, identify what might have been at the root of each example.

_____

_____

_____

_____

2. Discuss or consider Alicia's conclusion: "Sometimes we romanticize the early church, but they were no strangers to this type of spiritual pain."

_____

_____

_____

_____

_____

RESPOND

1. Are any of the examples of disillusionment within the community of faith listed on pages 190–191 familiar to you?

_____

_____

_____

_____

_____

2. If so, hold these examples up to God and ask Him to bring a new layer of healing to you through the upcoming chapters.

_____

_____

_____

_____

_____

GOD'S PEOPLE CAN BE CLUMSY, AND SOMETIMES EVEN CRUEL,
IN HANDLING ONE ANOTHER'S PAIN.

Chapter 40

· · ·

SUNDAY SCHOOLED

REFLECT

1. Write out the first of eleven encouragements in this section: When disillusioned with God's people . . .

2. What does Alicia identify as a frequent (but underestimated) contributor to pain in the family of God? Do you agree?

3. Share any recent personal examples that come to mind of you and someone you love sincerely seeing something differently from opposite sides of the same table.

FROM SIMON THE ZEALOT TO MATTHEW THE TAX COLLECTOR, FROM JAMES AND JOHN, SONS OF THUNDER, TO PETER THE ROCK, JESUS COLLECTED QUITE A COMBUSTIBLE CREW.

STUDY

Read John 13:34-35:

> "A new command I give you: Love one another. As I have loved you, so you must love one another. By this all men will know that you are my disciples, if you love one another."

Of this verse, Alicia states, "something of eternal weight—i.e., 'all men will know'—rested (and still rests) on what is sometimes referred to as the eleventh commandment" (page 193). How might our love for "one another" influence the eternity of "all"?

_____

_____

_____

_____

_____

_____

_____

_____

_____

_____

_____

_____

TRULY, TWO ARE BETTER THAN ONE. AND . . .
TWO ARE MORE COMPLICATED THAN ONE.

RESPOND

1. Draw a 6 in the space below. Then imagine Jesus seated facing you.

2. Ask Him if there are any areas in which He wants to help you see your life from His perspective.

AS WE LOSE ILLUSIONS AND GAIN REALITY ABOUT ONE ANOTHER, LOVE IS JESUS' CALL TO US. IT IS PURE AND PURIFYING, CHALLENGING AND DEATH-DEFYING.

Chapter 41

· · ·

LESS THAN BLESSED

REFLECT

1. Write out encouragement 2: When disillusioned with God's people . . .

   _____

   _____

2. When it comes to interpersonal pain in the body of Christ, which do you more often blame: shadows of sin or shadows of strength?

   _____

   _____

3. How might the concept of strength shadows help you navigate interpersonal disillusionment?

   _____

   _____

   _____

   _____

4. Either in a group or individually, walk through the exercise Alicia describes on pages 199–200.

   _____

   _____

   _____

   _____

5. Then share any discoveries you have made about yourself.

_____

_____

_____

_____

_____

_____

6. In your own words, how was Alicia's husband living in the shadow of her strengths? (See page 200.)

_____

_____

_____

_____

_____

7. Looking over the descriptions of producers, relaters, and thinkers on pages 201–202, how would you describe yourself?

_____

_____

_____

_____

_____

_____

> STRENGTH SHADOWS ARE A LESS INTUITIVE SOURCE OF DISILLUSIONMENT BECAUSE IT RARELY OCCURS TO US THAT OUR GIFTINGS COULD SUPPLY ANYTHING OTHER THAN BLESSING TO A RELATIONSHIP.

STUDY

Read the following "one another" verses.

> Be at peace with each other. (Mark 9:50)
> Be devoted to one another in brotherly love. (Romans 12:10)
> Honor one another above yourselves. (Romans 12:10)
> Stop passing judgment on one another. (Romans 14:13)
> Accept one another, then, just as Christ accepted you. (Romans 15:7)
> Have equal concern for each other. (1 Corinthians 12:25)
> Carry each other's burdens. (Galatians 6:2)
> In humility consider others better than yourselves. (Philippians 2:3)
> Bear with each other. (Colossians 3:13)
> Forgive whatever grievances you may have against one another. (Colossians 3:13)
> Do not slander one another. (James 4:11)
> Each one should use whatever gift he has received to serve others. (1 Peter 4:10)

Think of the strength shadows from those near you that you regularly walk in. Highlight or star any verses that might strengthen you when others' shadows are the source of your pain.

_____

_____

_____

_____

_____

_____

_____

PERHAPS WE CAN LAUGH A BIT MORE AND BLAME SIN A BIT LESS FOR THE CHALLENGES WE FACE AS A COMMUNITY. PLAIN OLD *LIFE* AND *STRENGTH SHADOWS* CONFIRM THE INNATE COMPLEXITY OF LIFE TOGETHER *BEFORE* ANYTHING ELSE EVEN ENTERS THE ROOM.

RESPOND

1. Write down your strengths, those strengths' shadows, and the names of those who live in the shadow of your strengths.

MY STRENGTH	ITS SHADOW	THOSE WHO LIVE IN THE SHADOW OF MY STRENGTH

2. Spend time in prayer for those you named.

Chapter 42

. . .

HOW WE HEAR

REFLECT

1. Write out encouragement 3: When disillusioned with God's people . . .

_____

_____

2. Offer examples to show your agreement or disagreement with the following statement: "Sacrificing quality for quickness, we are shouting louder, but fewer of us seem to feel *heard*" (page 205).

_____

_____

_____

_____

_____

_____

3. On pages 205–206, what four attributes of generous listening does Alicia describe?

_____

_____

_____

_____

_____

_____

STUDY

Read 1 Peter 1:22:

Love one another deeply, from the heart.

Share any stories that come to mind of people who loved you well by listening to you from their hearts.

_____
_____
_____
_____
_____
_____
_____
_____
_____
_____
_____
_____
_____
_____
_____
_____
_____
_____
_____
_____

RESPOND

1. On page 205, Alicia describes "mercenary" listening in which we hear for our own sake more than for others' sake. Fill in the blanks for a further description of such listening.

Mercenary listening . . .

Mines conversations for only what _____ _____.
Gathers information to _____ our side.
Selectively _____ through all the words to piece together evidence of our _____.
Listens to take, use, and to _____ instead of listening ____ _____ _____
to others and to ourselves.

2. In prayer, ask God to help you be a more generous listener.

_____

_____

_____

_____

_____

_____

_____

_____

_____

_____

GENEROUS LISTENING IS BECOMING A LOST ART.
PERHAPS BECAUSE LISTENING, IN GENERAL, HAS BECOME A
LOST SKILL. AS A CULTURE, WE NOW COLLECT INFORMATION
IN CLIPS AND BITS THAT ARE RARELY, IF EVER, CAPABLE OF
CAPTURING THE COMPLEXITIES OF A HUMAN HEART.

Chapter 43

. . .

HOLDING THE GLASS

REFLECT

1. Write out encouragement 4: When disillusioned with God's people . . .

2. How did the image of holding the glass relate to the story of Alicia's son?

3. In your own words, what is the difference between unknown, unstated, and unshared expectations? (See pages 208–209.)

4. Generate examples of each type of expectation.

5. Which do you feel causes the most spiritual pain in your relationships?

_____

_____

_____

_____

STUDY

Read Mark 9:33-35:

They came to Capernaum. When he was in the house, he asked them, "What were you arguing about on the road?" But they kept quiet because on the way they had argued about who was the greatest. Sitting down, Jesus called the Twelve and said, "If anyone wants to be first, he must be the very last, and the servant of all."

1. Add some context to this passage. What happened right before and right after these verses?

_____

_____

_____

2. What were the disciples arguing about?

_____

3. If studying with others, do a one-to-two-minute impromptu skit of what this might have sounded like.

4. How would you describe Jesus' response to their conversation?

_____

_____

5. Since Jesus didn't fire the guys for a lack of character, what do you think His expectations of them were at this point in their journey with Him?

_____

_____

6. What do you think His expectations are of you at this point in your journey?

_____

_____

_____

_____

RESPOND

1. Think of a difficult interpersonal relationship. What unmet expectations do you have?

_____

_____

_____

_____

_____

_____

_____

2. Ask God if you have been holding the glass of your expectations for that relationship too high, too low, or just right.

_____

_____

_____

_____

_____

_____

TAKING THE TIME TO IDENTIFY HOW HIGH ABOVE REALITY WE ARE HOLDING THE GLASSES OF OUR INTERPERSONAL EXPECTATIONS IS A WISE USE OF ENERGY, ESPECIALLY IN THE NIGHT.

Chapter 44

. . .

TABLE STRETCHES

REFLECT

1. Write out encouragement 5: When disillusioned with God's people . . .

_____

_____

_____

_____

2. What is the difference between mental flexibility and relativism?

_____

_____

_____

_____

3. Growing up, was mental flexibility emphasized in your family or community? If so, how? If not, why not?

_____

_____

_____

_____

_____

_____

4. Look back over the last ten years. As a culture, do you feel we have become more or less able to agree to disagree? Why?

_____

_____

_____

_____

5. Discuss the following quote: "We say we want feedback, but in practice, perhaps what we really want are thumbs-up and hearts. Our lack of mental flexibility is revoking our freedom to simply be honest" (page 212).

_____

_____

_____

_____

_____

_____

DISILLUSIONMENT IN THE COMMUNITY OF FAITH
IS NOT EVIDENCE OF FAILED RELATIONSHIPS.
IT IS EVIDENCE OF _EXISTING_ RELATIONSHIPS.

STUDY

Read Romans 12:10, 18

Be devoted to one another in brotherly love. Honor one another above yourselves. . . . If it is possible, as far as it depends on you, live at peace with everyone.

1. Rewrite this scriptural admonition from Paul to the believers in Rome.

_____

_____

_____

_____

2. Alicia speaks of how each generation values honesty and unity but not always in the same order. (See page 212.) In what ways have you seen different ordering of honesty and unity contribute to a lack of peace in the family of God?

_____

_____

_____

_____

_____

RESPOND

Picture yourself at God's table with someone you don't particularly enjoy. See God as your mutual Host. Then respond to Alicia's closing question: "Could I, should I, dare I make a case to Father God as to why this other soul should not be at His table in heaven? If not, then perhaps I should mentally stretch toward them a bit more here on earth" (page 213).

_____

_____

_____

_____

_____

_____

> WHILE WE EXPEND OUR ENERGY OVERREACTING TO ONE ANOTHER, THE TRULY GREAT COMMISSION GOD HAS ENTRUSTED TO US (SEE MATTHEW 28:18-20) GOES UNATTENDED.

• • •

Disillusionment with Others

A new command I give you: Love one another. As I have loved you,
so you must love one another. By this all men will know
that you are my disciples, if you love one another.

JOHN 13:34

Chapter 45

· · ·

TO HAVE, OR NOT
TO HAVE, A COW

REFLECT

1. Write out encouragement 6: When disillusioned with God's people . . .

   _____

   _____

2. In the opening story, how was the younger brother's response to his older brother's cow crisis "close to a textbook example of *differentiation*"? (See page 215.)

   _____

   _____

3. On a scale of 0 (never) to 10 (always), how strong is your tendency to take care of other people's cows?

   _____

   _____

4. "In the context of disillusionment with others, differentiation makes us less vulnerable to being manipulated by the power of others' emotions. Knowing where we end and others begin helps us find enough ground to stand upon and make decisions based on accuracy instead of felt urgency" (page 216). Do you agree or disagree? Why?

   _____

   _____

   _____

   _____

   _____

STUDY

Read Luke 23:8-15:

> When Herod saw Jesus, he was greatly pleased, because for a long time he had been wanting to see him. From what he had heard about him, he hoped to see him perform some miracle. He plied him with many questions, but Jesus gave him no answer. The chief priests and the teachers of the law were standing there, vehemently accusing him. Then Herod and his soldiers ridiculed and mocked him. Dressing him in an elegant robe, they sent him back to Pilate.

1. What tactics did Herod use to try to manipulate and control Jesus?

_____

_____

2. What would it have taken for you to be silent in the midst of such treatment?

_____

_____

_____

RESPOND

Bring a difficult relationship before God in prayer. Ask God to help you see where that person ends and you begin, to help you differentiate between *them and their emotions* and *you and your choices*.

_____

_____

_____

_____

_____

KNOWING WHERE WE END AND OTHERS BEGIN HELPS US FIND ENOUGH GROUND TO STAND UPON AND MAKE DECISIONS BASED ON ACCURACY INSTEAD OF FELT URGENCY.

Chapter 46

. . .

A MUSCULAR MERCY

REFLECT

1. Write out encouragement 7: When disillusioned with God's people . . .

_____

_____

2. "Speaking is not always the commission of seeing" (page 219). What other reasons might God have for giving you insight besides using your voice to correct what you see?

_____

_____

_____

_____

3. Alicia describes Jesus' rebukes as "surgical." (See page 220.) Why?

_____

_____

_____

4. List the four principles offered to guide speech that heals:

_____

_____

_____

_____

_____

5. How common do you think it is for believers to clothe correction in humor? (See page 220.)

_____

_____

_____

6. In what ways is the fourth principle—limiting your circle of advisers and sympathizers—both important and difficult in our digital age?

_____

_____

_____

_____

7. When looking for someone to confide in, what characteristics does Alicia encourage you to avoid? To pursue?

AVOID THOSE WHO . . .	SEARCH FOR THOSE WHO . . .

GOD, IN HIS LOVE, DOES NOT INSTANTLY TELL US EVERYTHING THAT IS TRUE ABOUT US. HE SEES MORE THAN HE SAYS. MERCY GUIDES BOTH HIS SPEECH AND HIS SILENCE.

STUDY

1. Read these additional "one another" verses.

> Instruct one another. (Romans 15:14)
> If you keep on biting and devouring each other . . . you will be destroyed by each other. (Galatians 5:15)
> Let us not become conceited, provoking and envying each other. (Galatians 5:26)
> Speak to one another with psalms, hymns and spiritual songs. (Ephesians 5:19)
> Encourage each other. (1 Thessalonians 4:18)
> Spur one another on toward love and good deeds. (Hebrews 10:24)
> Don't grumble against each other. (James 5:9)

2. From these verses, describe speech that heals instead of harms.

_____

_____

_____

_____

_____

_____

_____

RESPOND

Think of someone you'd like to tell a thing or two. Ask yourself why you want to speak, and consider the possibilities listed on page 220: "For good? For God? To vent? To purge? To avenge? To save face?"

_____

_____

_____

_____

_____

_____

Chapter 47

. . .

WHAT WAS, WAS

REFLECT

1. Write out encouragement 8: When disillusioned with God's people . . .

_____

_____

_____

2. Consider or discuss the following statement: "Lies have no healing power. Yet how often do we go back and change the facts? How often do we spin the beginning to fabricate some sort of pseudo-peace about the end? Deception cannot resolve disillusionment" (page 224).

_____

_____

_____

_____

3. Recall an example of revisionism from your own life. What reasoning helped you justify a rewrite of the true story?

_____

_____

_____

_____

_____

STUDY

Read John 8:31-32:

> To the Jews who had believed him, Jesus said, "If you hold to my teaching, you are really my disciples. Then you will know the truth, and the truth will set you free."

1. Speaking to believers, Jesus said that through His teachings, they would know truth, and through truth, they would know freedom. Discuss this verse alongside the following quote: "An unresolved mystery is far safer for our souls than anesthetizing our minds with untruth" (page 225).

   _____

   _____

   _____

   _____

   _____

2. Since untruth can't heal, what motivates us to hold fast to it?

   _____

   _____

   _____

   _____

   _____

   _____

   _____

   _____

WHEN WE ARE DISILLUSIONED, IT IS EXTREMELY EASY TO FALL INTO A HURT-FUELED (INSTEAD OF FACT-FUELED) FORM OF REVISIONISM IN WHICH WE REWRITE THE PAST IN ORDER TO MAKE SENSE OF THE PRESENT.

RESPOND

"When disillusioned, remember that painful endings do not have the authority to void miraculous beginnings" (page 225). Allow these words to sink into your heart. Be attentive to any revisionism God wants to address in your memory.

Chapter 48

• • •

THE "SHOW ME" STATE

REFLECT

1. Write out encouragement 9: When disillusioned with God's people . . .

   _____

   _____

2. Upon what reasoning does Alicia base this encouragement? (See page 227.)

   _____

   _____

   _____

3. Recount Alicia's unusual experience regarding Joel 2:23-27.

   _____

   _____

   _____

   _____

4. Reading Joel in the midst of that interpersonal pain shifted Alicia's understanding of her assignment. In what way? (See pages 228–229.)

   _____

   _____

   _____

   _____

   _____

STUDY

Read Joel 2:12-13:

"Even now," declares the LORD, "return to me with all your heart, with fasting and weeping and mourning." Rend your heart and not your garments. Return to the LORD your God, for he is gracious and compassionate, slow to anger and abounding in love, and he relents from sending calamity.

1. As an evil enemy came against them, what response did God ask for from His people?

   _____

   _____

2. Why is this encouragement to "stay teachable" especially difficult when we see ourselves as the less guilty part of the tango?

   _____

   _____

   _____

RESPOND

"This encouragement to remain teachable when disillusioned with God's people is based in certainty that God does not waste anything here on earth" (page 227). Breathe a prayer of faith: "God, I trust You to not waste this pain. Grant me eyes to see *treasures of darkness.*" (See Isaiah 45:3.)

_____

_____

_____

_____

> EVERY DISILLUSIONMENT CONTAINS WITHIN IT THE OPPORTUNITY FOR HEARTS AND LOVE TO BE PURIFIED BY GOD. BUT IN ORDER FOR THAT TO HAPPEN, WE MUST WORK TO REMAIN TEACHABLE WHEN WRONGED AND HUMBLE WHEN IN THE RIGHT.

Chapter 49

. . .

FROM ABOVE

REFLECT

1. Write out encouragement 10: When disillusioned with God's people . . .

_____

_____

2. "It is one thing to love the community of faith when we think it is perfect. It is quite another thing to love the community of faith when we know it is not" (page 230). Consider the different generations represented in your community of faith. Do you notice any differences in the resilience of their commitment to the gathered body of Christ? If so, what factors might have contributed to this difference?

_____

_____

_____

_____

3. Think of the strongest, healthiest marriage you have personally observed. Surely, they could not see into the future when they stood at an altar together and said, "I do." What practices or attitudes have helped them stay true to one another as they journeyed through the (sometimes painful) gaining of reality about each other year after year?

_____

_____

_____

_____

_____

4. Alicia suggests that the type of love Jesus called us to isn't a feeling but a choice. (See pages 231–232.) In the context of the community of faith, do you think love is really love when it lacks lovely emotions?

_____

_____

_____

5. Name and describe the two types of "love" God called Alicia to avoid when she was disillusioned with His people. (See pages 232–233.)

_____

_____

_____

_____

STUDY

Read 1 John 4:19-21:

We love because he first loved us. If anyone says, "I love God," yet hates his brother, he is a liar. For anyone who does not love his brother, whom he has seen, cannot love God, whom he has not seen. And he has given us this command: Whoever loves God must also love his brother.

1. According to John, is it possible to love God and hate His people?

_____

_____

_____

ONE OF THE REASONS OUR ABILITY TO LOVE GROWS STRONGER THROUGH EVERY CYCLE OF DISILLUSIONMENT WITH GOD'S PEOPLE IS BECAUSE, AS WE LOSE ILLUSIONS, OUR CHOICE TO KEEP LOVING OCCURS IN THE CONTEXT *OF GREATER ACCURACY.*

2. Jesus called John a "Son of Thunder" (see Mark 3:17). How do you think John journeyed from being a hotheaded, judgmental follower who wanted to call down fire on Samaritans (see Luke 9:54) to being known today as the apostle of love?

_____

_____

_____

_____

RESPOND

"Jesus loved the disciples *accurately*. He knew who they really were, but His love was not sourced in their behavior. Then and now, Jesus' love flows *from above*. This is how we can love people we do not like" (page 231). In prayer, ask God to help you love people you do not like.

_____

_____

_____

_____

_____

_____

_____

_____

ATTEMPTING TO CORRECT EMOTION BY ADDING
MORE EMOTION IS RARELY EFFECTIVE. YET HOW OFTEN
DO WE RESPOND TO OTHERS' ANXIETY BY BECOMING ANXIOUS?
HOW OFTEN DO WE REACT TO OTHERS' STRESS BY
BECOMING STRESSED? IT IS LIKE ADDING FUEL TO A FIRE
AND WONDERING WHY IT DOES NOT GO OUT.

Chapter 50

. . .

FORTY-FOUR
CHAPTERS PAST BAIL

REFLECT

1. What was your first response when you read, "In the roughly sixty 'one another' and 'each other' New Testament verses that instruct us on life together, we are told to love one another well over a dozen times, yet we are not told to trust each other even once." (page 234).

_____

_____

_____

_____

_____

2. In your own words, what is the difference between love and trust? (See page 235.)

_____

_____

_____

_____

3. Why is this distinction important when navigating pain in the family of God?

_____

_____

_____

_____

4. Write out encouragement 11: When disillusioned with God's people . . .

_____

_____

5. Alicia states that "David did not surrender to Saul's sickness. David did not self-martyr on Saul's spears. David left" (page 236). How is this type of departure different from bailing?

_____

_____

_____

_____

_____

STUDY

Read 1 Samuel 26, excerpts of which are below:

David set out and went to the place where Saul had camped. He saw where Saul and Abner son of Ner, the commander of the army, had lain down. (26:5)

Abishai said to David, "Today God has delivered your enemy into your hands. Now let me pin him to the ground with one thrust of my spear; I won't strike him twice." But David said to Abishai, "Don't destroy him!" (26:8-9)

"The LORD forbid that I should lay a hand on the LORD's anointed. Now get the spear and water jug that are near his head, and let's go." (26:11)

Then David crossed over to the other side and stood on top of the hill some distance away; there was a wide space between them. (26:13)

Saul recognized David's voice and said, "Is that your voice, David my son?" David replied, "Yes it is, my lord the king." And he added, "Why is my lord pursuing his servant? What have I done, and what wrong am I guilty of?" (26:17-18)

Then Saul said, "I have sinned. Come back, David my son." (26:21)

Then Saul said to David, "May you be blessed, my son David; you will do great things and surely triumph." So David went on his way, and Saul returned home. (26:25)

Throughout this story, trace the dual threads of how David loved Saul but did not trust Saul. Have you ever loved someone that you did not trust? If so, describe any confusion you experienced in navigating your way through that relationship.

_____

_____

_____

_____

_____

_____

_____

RESPOND

"When we find ourselves in similar relationships, like David, we hope that 'Saul' gets better. We pray for 'Saul's' deliverance. But sometimes we need to hope and pray from a distance" (page 237). Offer prayers from a distance for the Sauls in your life.

_____

_____

_____

_____

_____

_____

_____

_____

> LOVE IS SOMETHING *GIVEN*. TRUST IS SOMETHING *EARNED*.
> LOVE IS ABOUT *GENEROSITY*. TRUST IS ABOUT *SAFETY*.
> TREATING THE TWO AS SYNONYMS CAN BE DISASTROUS.

Chapter 51

. . .

THE MAN IN THE MIDDLE

REFLECT

1. Which of the encouragements for navigating disillusionment with God's people (see pages 239–240) was the most surprising for you?

2. Which might be the most challenging for you to implement?

3. "Yes, Barnabas and Paul parted ways. And God went with Paul. And God went with Barnabas" (page 241). Do you have any similar stories? If so, close your eyes and picture God going with you *and* God going with the other person. Then share any responses you have to the image.

4. Consider reading aloud the following declaration and prayer of commitment as a group or with someone you love:

We refuse to abandon each other.
We will stand together with our strengths and shadows, successes and failures.
We make this commitment not for commitment's sake, nor for our sake,
but because our Savior is committed to us and
He has committed us to one another.

Spirit, make us one. Help us answer the prayer of Jesus
so that by our love all men will know
that we are disciples of the one true God.
Strengthen us to declare in one voice:
"There is a living God. Jesus is His name.
He died so we could live and lives to guide us home.
Together we invite you into the safety of God's existence, forgiveness, and love."

STUDY

Read John 17:20-23:

"My prayer is not for them alone. I pray also for those who will believe in me through their message, that all of them may be one, Father, just as you are in me and I am in you. May they also be in us so that the world may believe that you have sent me. I have given them the glory that you gave me, that they may be one as we are one: I in them and you in me. May they be brought to complete unity to let the world know that you sent me and have loved them even as you have loved me."

1. In this passage, underline the "why" Jesus identified in His request for His followers to be one.

2. Brainstorm ways you can contribute to answering Jesus' prayer in your generation.

_____

_____

_____

_____

_____

_____

RESPOND

Quiet your heart before God. Below, write out a prayer asking God for the strength to commit to His body on this earth until seeing Him face-to-face makes loving those who have hurt you much easier.

_____

_____

_____

_____

_____

_____

_____

_____

> WHEN WE ARE DISILLUSIONED, IT CAN SEEM AS THOUGH GOD HAS HIS BACK TO US. BUT SPIRITUALLY, WHAT IS REALLY HAPPENING IS THAT GOD IS FACING OFF WHAT HAS COME AGAINST US. HE IS THE MAN IN THE MIDDLE OF ALL OUR INTERPERSONAL PAIN IN THE FAITH FAMILY.

Chapter 52

· · ·

CONCLUSION

REFLECT

1. Looking back over all the encouragements and principles Alicia offered, what stands out to you as something you never want to forget from your study of *The Night Is Normal*?

_____

_____

_____

_____

_____

2. If you could ask Alicia one question, what would it be?

_____

_____

_____

3. "Every time you choose to follow Jesus in the night, your faith grows and you build momentum to keep following Him in the days (and decades) to come" (page 243). Write down the three steps we often take when we are following someone but have no idea where they are going (see page 244):

_____

_____

_____

_____

4. Pray for or with those near you. Ask God to strengthen them to keep following Him through every day and every night.

_____

_____

_____

_____

STUDY

Read John 14:3-5:

"If I go and prepare a place for you, I will come back and take you to be with me that you also may be where I am. You know the way to the place where I am going." Thomas said to him, "Lord, we don't know where you are going, so how can we know the way?" Jesus answered, "I am the way and the truth and the life. No one comes to the Father except through me."

1. What did Thomas think he needed from Jesus?

_____

2. What did Jesus offer him?

_____

_____

3. Tradition holds that in AD 72, Thomas was martyred in India for sharing the good news about Jesus. It would seem that Jesus' directions proved sufficient for Thomas to find his way Home. In what ways has Jesus' "Follow me" already guided you into difficult days?

_____

_____

_____

_____

4. Prayerfully, recommit to the sufficiency of Jesus as your Way, Truth, and Life.

_____

_____

_____

_____

_____

_____

_____

_____

_____

> FOLLOWING JESUS IS THE SELF-SUSTAINING CORE
> OF COMMITMENT AND THE NOT-SO-CRYPTIC KEY TO
> SPIRITUAL GROWTH THROUGH DISILLUSIONMENT.

RESPOND

1. Reflect on the story Alicia shared about the father whose grip around his son's wrist carried him to safety when, in fear, the son let go of his dad's pinkie. (See pages 245–246.)

_____

_____

_____

_____

_____

2. As you turn the final page in this study, thank God for His mercy through the nights of faith and declare this ancient truth aloud:

> You, O LORD, keep my lamp burning;
> my God turns my darkness into light.
>
> PSALM 18:28

ABOUT THE AUTHOR

As a speaker, leadership mentor, and award-winning writer, Dr. Alicia Britt Chole places words like an artist applying paint to a canvas. Nothing is wasted. Every word matters. Heads and hearts are equally engaged. A former atheist, Alicia's worldview was interrupted by Jesus as she began her university studies. Of that experience Alicia states, "I would have had to commit emotional and intellectual suicide to deny God's reality." Today, her raw faith and love for God's Word hold the attention of saints and skeptics alike. Alicia focuses on less than trendy topics like spiritual pain, the leader's soul, the potential of anonymous years, decrease as a discipline, and the abuse of authority. Business leaders, pastors, college students, and churches agree: Alicia is an unusually disarming combination of realism and hope, intellect and grace, humor and art. Alicia and Barry have been married for thirty years. Along with their three amazing children (all Choles through the miracle of adoption), they live in the country off of a dirt road in the Ozarks. Alicia holds a doctorate in leadership and spiritual formation from George Fox Evangelical Seminary and is the founding director and lead mentor of Leadership Investment Intensives, Inc., a nonprofit devoted to providing confidential and customized soul-care to leaders in the marketplace and church. Her favorite things include thunderstorms, honest questions, LOTR, and anything with jalapeños. In a culture obsessed with things new and countable, Alicia brings ancient truth to life. Visit Alicia online at www.aliciachole.com and on Instagram @aliciabrittchole.

NOTES

NOTES

NOTES

Though faith shines in the full sun, it grows depth in the dark.

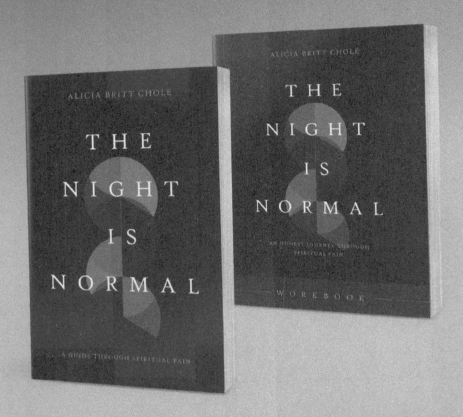